ETHICS AND LAW
in DENTAL HYGIENE

ETHICS AND LAW

in DENTAL HYGIENE

FOURTH EDITION

Kristin Minihan-Anderson, *RDH, MSDH*

Clinical Dental Hygienist
Adjunct Faculty
University of New Haven
West Haven, Connecticut

ELSEVIER

Elsevier
3251 Riverport Lane
St. Louis, Missouri 63043

ETHICS AND LAW IN DENTAL HYGIENE FOURTH EDITION

Notice

Practitioners and researchers must always rely on their own experience and knowledge in evaluating and using any information, methods, compounds or experiments described herein. Because of rapid advances in the medical sciences, in particular, independent verification of diagnoses and drug dosages should be made. To the fullest extent of the law, no responsibility is assumed by Elsevier, authors, editors or contributors for any injury and/or damage to persons or property as a matter of products liability, negligence or otherwise, or from any use or operation of any methods, products, instructions, or ideas contained in the material herein.

Previous editions copyrighted 2017, 2010, and 2002.

International Standard Book Number: 978-0-323-76119-2

Senior Content Strategist: Kelly Skelton
Senior Content Development Manager: Somodatta Roy Choudhury
Senior Content Development Specialist: Shilpa Kumar
Production Manager: Deena Burgess
Senior Project Manager: Anne Collett
Design Direction: Renee Duenow
Marketing Manager: Joshua Caparas

Printed in India

Last digit is the print number: 9 8 7 6 5 4 3 2 1

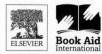

Working together
to grow libraries in
developing countries

www.elsevier.com • www.bookaid.org

Contributors

Phyllis L. Beemsterboer, RDH, EdD

Professor Emeritus
School of Dentistry
Oregon Health & Science University
Portland, Oregon
Associate Director
Center for Ethics in Health Care
Oregon Health & Science University
Portland, Oregon

Linda D. Boyd, MS, EdD

Associate Dean, Professor
Forsyth School of Dental Hygiene
Massachusetts College or Pharmacy & Health Sciences
Boston, Massachusetts

Michele P. Carr, BS, MA, EdE(c)

Associate Professor Emeritus
Dental Hygiene
The Ohio State University
Columbus, Ohio

Frank Catalanotto, DMD

Community Dentist and Behavioral Science
College of Dentistry
University of Florida
Gainesville, Florida

Gary Chiodo, DMD

Professor and Dean
School of Dentistry
University of Washington
Seattle, Washington

Matt Crespin, MPH, RDH

Executive Director
Children's Health Alliance of Wisconsin
Milwaukee, Wisconsin

Laura Fassacesia, RDH, BSDH, MSDH

2nd-year Clinic Coordinator
Professor of Periodontology & Oral Pathology
Plaza College Dental Hygiene Program
Forest Hills, New York

Deirdre M. Fiorini, MSDH, RDH

Professor
Dental Hygiene
Plaza College
Forest Hills, New York

Shavonne R. Healy, MSDH, RDH

Contributor
Dental Hygiene
Fones School of Dental Hygiene
Bridgeport, Connecticut

Monica L. Hospenthal, RDH, BS, MEd

Director
Dental Hygiene
Pierce College Fort Steilacoom
Lakewood, Washington

Donna Lesser, RDH, EdD

Retired Educator, Consultant

Kristin Minihan-Anderson, RDH, MSDH

Clinical Dental Hygienist
Adjunct Faculty
Dental Hygiene
University of New Haven
West Haven, Connecticut

Pamela Overman, BS, MS, EdD

Professor Emerita
School of Dentistry
University of Missouri-Kansas City
Kansas City, Missouri

David Ozar, PhD
Professor Emeritus
Philosophy
Loyola University Chicago
Chicago, Illinois

Toni M. Roucka, RN, DDS, MA
Associate Professor and Associate Dean for Academic Affairs
Restorative Dentistry
University of Illinois Chicago
Chicago, Illinois

Alexandra D. E. Sheppard, RDH, BA, DipDH, MEd
Clinical Professor
Dentistry
University of Alberta
Edmonton, Alberta, Canada

Sandra Stramoski, RDH, MSDH
Associate Professor
Dental Hygiene
University of Bridgeport
Bridgeport, Connecticut

Karen S. Williams, BS, MS
Associate Professor
Dental Hygiene
University of Bridgeport
Bridgeport, Connecticut

Pamela Zarkowski, JD, MPH
Provost and Vice President for Academic Affairs
University of Detroit Mercy
Detroit, Michigan
Professor
Practice Essentials and Interprofessional Education
University of Detroit Mercy School of Dentistry
Detroit, Michigan

Reviewers

Lezlie M. Cantrell, RDH, BSDH, MSDH, PhD
Associate Professor
Dental Hygiene
Missouri Southern State University
Joplin, Missouri

April Catlett, PhD, MDH, BHSA, RDH, EDA
Program Chair
Dental Hygiene
Central Georgia Technical College Pomona
Warner Robins, Georgia

Tammy S. Clossen, RDH, BS, MS, PhD
Assistant Professor
Dental Hygiene
Pennsylvania College of Technology
Williamsport, Pennsylvania

Kathleen Feres-Patry, RDH, Dip DH, BEd
Ethics & Jurisprudence Educator, Privacy Officer
Canadian National Institute of Health (CNIH)
Ottawa, Ontario, Canada

Brenda H. Fisher, RDH, BSDH
Associate Program Director
Dental Hygiene
Asheville-Buncombe Technical Community College
Asheville, North Carolina

Lisa Graciana, RDH, EdM
Associate Professor
Dental Hygiene
Rock Valley College
Rockford, Illinois

Kristin M. Hofer, RDH, MSDH
Assistant Professor
Dental Hygiene
SUNY Broome Community College
Binghamton, New York
Adjunct Professor
Dental Hygiene
University of Bridgeport
Bridgeport, Connecticut

Christine Patel, RDH, BSDH, MA
Associate Professor and Instructor-in-Charge
Dental Hygiene
St. Petersburg College
St. Petersburg, Florida

Cynthia Senior, RDH, BS, MEd
Assistant Professor and Clinic Director
Department of Dental Hygiene
University of Mississippi Medical Center School of
   Dentistry
Jackson, Mississippi

Ancillary Writers

CASE STUDIES

Christine Nathe, RDH, MS
Professor and Director
Division of Dental Hygiene
Vice Chair
Department of Dental Medicine
University of New Mexico
Albuquerque, New Mexico

TEST BANK

Jennifer Zabel, MS, BS, RDH, CDA
Developer
Senior Allied Health Program
MedCerts (A Stride Company)
Livonia, Michigan

This book is dedicated to my sons,
Cody John and Colton Robert Anderson,
and my granddaughters,
Charlee Rae and Callie Rose Anderson.
May I always make you proud.

To Peter L. Bonagura,
for his undying support, encouragement, and love,
all of which mean more to me than words could ever express.

To my mentor and dear friend, Olga A.C. Ibsen,
who inspires me to believe I can achieve the unthinkable
professionally and personally.

Preface

When Alfred Civilion Fones graduated from dental school in 1890, he went home to Bridgeport, Connecticut, to practice dentistry with his father, also a dentist. The overwhelming majority of patients treated within their practice required the extraction of decayed teeth.

Dr. Fones was convinced that if the public were educated about how to prevent dental disease, fewer would require treatment resulting from the progression of disease. Furthermore, Dr. Fones understood that oral and systemic health were inextricably linked, requiring the need for a distinct profession within dentistry focused on prevention and oral health education.

Irene E. Newman, Dr. Fones's dental assistant and cousin, began to provide dental hygiene services within his practice in 1907. Undeterred by the ridicule of his peers, in 1913 Dr. Fones, with the help of Irene Newman, opened the first school of dental hygiene and began teaching the first class of dental hygienists, with Irene Newman receiving the first dental hygiene license in the world in 1917 from the State of Connecticut. His vision was for dental hygienists to provide education and preventive care where the public was easily accessed, such as public schools, public clinics, and institutions, in addition to private dental practices.

The profession of dental hygiene has evolved tremendously from its inception, as have the needs of the public. The complexity of cases treated and work settings within which dental hygienists practice creates the need for a resource targeting the potential ethical dilemmas and legal liability these professionals encounter on a daily basis.

Background and Importance to the Profession

It is essential for dental hygienists to understand and appreciate the ethical and legal obligations faced in the provision of care to the public.

Audience

This textbook provides content related to ethics and law as they apply to the practice of dental hygiene. Within this fourth edition of *Ethics and Law in Dental Hygiene*, future and current dental hygiene professionals can benefit from not just the coverage of ethics and law but also the relevant connections between the two.

Organization

This textbook is organized into three sections, with the first two sections focusing on content and the third devoted to application. The first section begins with the topic of risk management, presents the foundational aspects of ethics, and introduces an ethical decision-making tool for the analysis of ethical dilemmas. Legal concepts are discussed in the second section and provide information on state practice acts, an overview of the legal system, and the dental hygienist's relationship with the patient and employer.

The third section provides 30 case scenarios for the reader to discuss and analyze that are authored by various contributors with expertise in their respective content areas. Questions are provided to stimulate thought and discussion, including opportunity to use the ethical decision-making model to work through dilemmas proposed in case studies. The cases are hypothetical, providing a range of materials to facilitate meaningful discussion, and the situations presented are relevant to those experienced in dentistry and dental hygiene.

Ten "testlets" are also included to help prepare students for the National Board Dental Hygiene Examination (NBDHE). (A testlet is a short clinical scenario with a series of associated test items that focus on critical thinking and problem-solving skills.) Last, a listing of suggested activities and projects helps expand upon the topics presented in the textbook and encourages additional thought and discussion.

Key Features

- Coverage of ethics and law and how they apply to risk management.
- Concepts are discussed in the context of real-world relevance to help readers apply the knowledge to daily situations.
- A six-step decision-making model provides the framework to allow readers to take on ethical situations.
- Contributors include educators, administrators, and clinicians who are renowned leaders in their respective fields of ethics, dentistry, and dental hygiene.
- Readers can sharpen their ethical and legal decision-making skills using the multitude of case studies covering a wide range of situations.

New to This Edition

- The topic of risk management has been moved to the beginning of the textbook and vastly expanded upon to provide context regarding why dental hygienists must possess a deep knowledge of the ethical and legal obligations associated with daily practice. Discussion of the Standards of Care related to dental hygiene help to emphasize the inextricable link between ethics and law.
- Returning chapters are revised, with expanded coverage of content related to the current practice of dental hygiene.
- Many new case studies have been provided by experts within a variety of dental and dental hygiene settings as well as ethics. These allow the reader to apply concepts learned throughout the textbook. Returning case studies have been revised and updated.
- "Testlets" have been revised and are available to encourage critical thinking, challenge problem-solving skills, and help students prepare for the National Board Dental Hygiene Exam (NBDHE).
- For instructors, the Evolve Resources website provides teaching resources, case study answers and rationales, and access to a test bank utilizing NBDHE format questions with answers. All have been updated to correspond with this edition of the textbook.
- For students, the Evolve Resources website includes practice quizzes and new case studies for additional studying.

Future and current dental hygiene professionals will find *Ethics and Law in Dental Hygiene*, 4th edition, to be a valuable resource as they navigate the complexities presented in the provision of care.

Acknowledgments

Many of us in dental hygiene education have used this textbook as an invaluable resource as we teach future dental hygienists how to navigate the ethical and legal obligations related to the practice of dental hygiene.

Phyllis L. Beemsterboer created this textbook to meet the need for content related to ethics and law specifically for the profession of dental hygiene. Her vision, knowledge, and passion have been the driving force behind the success of this textbook.

I would like to express my deepest gratitude to Phyllis for entrusting me with the responsibility of bringing forward the fourth edition of this textbook. It is my hope that this edition meets the benchmark she has set for this subject matter.

To say the collaborators for this textbook are renowned in their disciplines would be an understatement. Phyllis Beemsterboer and David Ozar are bioethics experts who have shared their knowledge to create the ethics section. Frank Catalanotto leads the discussion of social responsibility, discussing emerging provider models such as dental therapists and landmark government publications and initiatives related to access to care. All aspects of the law section of this textbook were provided by Pamela Zarkowski and Michele Carr. Pam, a lawyer, and Michele, a professor of dental hygiene, are experts in the laws governing the practice of dental hygiene. I am humbled to be associated with these incredible professionals.

A special thank you and acknowledgment goes to the contributors who provided case studies for this edition. Their contributions are greatly appreciated and help provide a method to apply the concepts presented in this textbook in a relevant way.

It truly takes a village to bring forward a textbook such as this. Thank you to everyone involved. Dental hygienists, current and future, will benefit from our efforts.

Kristin Minihan-Anderson

Contents

SECTION I

Ethics

is measured for the seriousness of the potential outcome and the likelihood of its occurrence. A strategy is then created to manage the risk in such a way as to minimize it or, in some cases, to eliminate it altogether.

Risk management programs generally focus on operational safety and compliance, product and equipment safety, and quality assurance.[1] The focus of operational safety and compliance programs is to maintain a safe environment for personnel, patients, and others to function, as well as compliance with applicable standards of care, regulations, guidelines, and recommendations from agencies such as the following:

- U.S. Department of Labor (DOL) Occupational Safety and Health Administration (OSHA)
  - Bloodborne Pathogens and Needlestick Prevention
- U.S. Department of Health & Human Services (HHS) Health Information Privacy
  - The Health Insurance Portability and Accountability Act of 1996 (HIPAA) requirements for protected health information and patient confidentiality
- HHS Centers for Disease Control and Prevention (CDC)
  - Infection Prevention Practices in Dental Settings

For this discussion, it is important to provide context regarding the terms *standards of care* and *regulations*. Standards of care are established by a profession and set the expectations of the provider–patient relationship. They are basically a set of expectations—or standards—describing the level of skill and care a reasonably competent and prudent provider should exhibit and, in turn, can be expected of all providers in a similar situation. If a provider deviates from the standards of care, exposure to liability and litigation may result, resulting in the provider being named as a defendant.

Typically, during malpractice litigation, the judge and jury require technical information from an expert in the field. Expert witnesses provide testimony regarding and opinions about the incident by reviewing the patient record, the outcomes, and whether or not the care provided met the acceptable standards of care.

Regulations are defined as a rule or order issued by an executive authority or regulatory agency of a government and having the force of law.[3] These are laws and are enforceable if not followed. These concepts will be discussed in depth in Chapters 8, 9, and 10.

Product and equipment safety programs ensure that personnel are updated regarding the safe use, storage, and maintenance of current products, materials, and equipment utilized within the practice.[1] *Quality assurance* programs evaluate and seek to improve processes and outcomes of patient care.

It is imperative that anyone charged with creating and implementing a risk management program in a dental setting possesses knowledge of the standards of care and scope of practice for the various providers employed by the practice, CDC infection prevention and control protocols, and OSHA and HIPAA requirements. In addition to enhanced patient and dental healthcare provider (DHCP) safety, effective risk management education combined with competent practice help to reduce allegations of malpractice and litigation.[1] According to the National Practitioner Data Bank, between the years 2011 and 2021 28,573 Adverse Action and Medical Malpractice Payment Reports involved dentists and 4406 were reported for dental hygienists and dental assistants.[2] All DHCPs have a vested interest in adhering to a risk management program.

Risk Identification

DHCPs encounter legal, ethical, and safety risks through daily interactions with the public and the completion of job-related tasks. The development of well-targeted procedures for minimizing adverse outcomes requires an awareness of the most frequently occurring negative incidents. Familiarity with the professional literature can support the dental hygienist in anticipating possible undesired situations that can occur most frequently in a dental practice. The literature shows that one of the primary reasons dental providers are sued in a court of law is failure to diagnose and/or treat disease. An assessment of a practice's policies and procedures (P&P) manual, including standard operating procedures, should be conducted and followed by a comparison to current standards related to facility operations, administration, personnel training, patient care, and scopes of practice to determine if updates are needed. A clear understanding of the risk exposure of a practice setting provides an opportunity for targeted problem-solving and corrective actions necessary to improve safety, patient care outcomes, and protection from legal liability.

A system of incident reporting provides valuable information during the risk identification process by pinpointing specific deficiencies in existing processes. This requires members of the dental team to complete a report for all adverse events or unusual incidents. Reporting may include issues related to patient care, patient complaints, and standard negligence such as "slip and fall" incidents. Occupational exposure by personnel to bloodborne pathogens and other potentially infectious material (OPIM) must also be reported. Such a report should focus on the concise recounting of facts rather than subjective assessments and should provide details of the event, including who, what, where, when, and why. These reports should not be retained in the patient record but, rather, maintained in a risk management portfolio. An incident reporting system permits the systematic tracking of adverse events.

As part of the risk identification process, a formalized **quality assurance program** that results in an improvement in the quality of patient care and overall organizational functioning should be implemented. The purpose of a quality assurance program is to assess patient care–related operations and administration of the practice setting as well as the delivery of patient care. This should be done systematically and continuously through the collection and analysis of reliable information, as described previously. The quality assurance process is an ongoing evaluation system that focuses on patterns of behavior rather than on isolated instances of behavior (i.e., incident reporting). It is a mechanism for assessing the quality of care and implementing and evaluating changes in the patient care delivery system to maintain or improve the quality of care.

In 1966, Avedis Donabedian published a groundbreaking paper titled *Evaluating the Quality of Medical Care*.[3] The Donabedian model describes *three dimensions* that provide the framework for healthcare quality measurement by which quality assurance programs can be modeled. A quality assurance program should include the assessment of these three dimensions of healthcare delivery: structure, process, and outcome (Box 1.1). The structure dimension considers components that contribute to the delivery of care such as administration, products and equipment, personnel, and facilities. The process dimension considers issues related to the delivery of clinical patient care, such as the process of care, standards of care, technical skill, and timeliness of care. The outcomes dimension considers the result of care, such as improvements in the health status and oral health literacy of patients as well as patient satisfaction. When risks are identified and quality is assessed in these domains,

• BOX 1.1	Dimensions of Quality Assessment

Structure	**Process**	**Outcomes**
Structures that contribute to the delivery of care	*The delivery of clinical care*	*Outcomes of care, health status, and behavior of patients*
Organization and administration	Process of care (assessment, dental hygiene diagnosis, planning, implementation, and evaluation: ADPIE)	Oral health improvement
Products and equipment		General health improvement
Personnel		Patient satisfaction
Facility	Technical skill	
	Timeliness of care	

improvement can be expected regarding patient care and patient and DHCP, safety which ultimately provides protection from liability. Identifying risks related to the three quality assessment domains can be accomplished using a risk assessment form such as the one provided in Box 1.2.[4] The results provide an opportunity to create a formal quality assurance process to address the problems identified.

The first step in a quality assurance process is the assessment of quality in one or more of the dimensions of healthcare delivery. The practice's P&P manual provides detailed instructions outlining processes that can be used to create an assessment checklist that identifies evaluation criteria applicable to the process to be assessed. The individual tasked with this job will use the checklist to collect data, analyze data, report results, and respond to results. Errors can be categorized according to severity (critical, noncritical, or minor) and handled accordingly.

A critical error is any error in a patient record that has the potential to adversely impact patient safety or alter care or treatment; noncritical errors impact document integrity but do not have the potential to alter patient safety, care, or treatment and do not alter the author's intended meaning. Minor errors have no impact on patient safety or care and do not diminish the integrity of the document.[5] The next step is to design and implement strategies intended to improve the quality of the healthcare delivery system. The final step is to evaluate the effect of these strategies on improving and maintaining quality. Quality assurance is a continuous, cyclic process of assessment, planning, implementation, and evaluation.

• BOX 1.3 **Components of the Patient Record**

The patient record should contain the following current and historical items:

- Signed acknowledgment of HIPAA policies
- Signed patient bill of rights and responsibilities
- Health history: current and past
- Clinical assessments: current and past
- Exams of head, neck, oral cavity, hard tissue, and periodontal charts
- Diagnostic radiographs, intra-/extraoral images, all diagnostic imaging and tests, study models, risk assessment findings, and dental hygiene diagnosis
- Planned treatment with signed informed consent and refusal forms
- Treatments and services rendered
- Communication with other healthcare providers
- Objective record of patient communication and interactions: telephone calls, emails, text messages, prescriptions, referrals, canceled/failed appointments, noncompliance with recommendations

jargon not identified in a formal documentation protocol should be avoided. A simple note such as "prophy" is not appropriate because it does not convey what procedures were performed, what products were used, or how the patient responded to treatment and patient education. A description of all treatment provided is required, including materials, products, and medicaments, when applicable.[15] Documentation should be completed by the provider of the care and completed in a timely manner following the patient visit as delaying the entry may cause incomplete and inaccurate documentation due to confusion with information about other patients treated that day. To ensure continuity of care it is essential that all providers adhere to the documentation protocols outlined in the P&P manual—any other provider should be able to review the patient record and easily continue the patient's treatment.[15] Additionally, healthcare providers must recognize the importance of confidentiality and guard this special trust and the patient's protected health information (PHI), which is both an ethical and legal requirement.

The patient record is not simply the documentation mentioned previously—it also includes radiographs, intraoral and extraoral images, three-dimensional scans, study models, referrals made to and reports back from other healthcare providers, and results of diagnostic tests. A patient may request that a copy of his or her record be transferred to another provider; a signed formal release-of-records document should be obtained. A dental office may charge a reasonable fee to duplicate the records and forward them—however, withholding the transfer of records because of lack of receiving a fee is not legally permitted.

Most patient records are created electronically using a practice management software program. These programs automatically record a date-and-time stamp for entries, identify the provider entering the information, and track any changes to existing data. A records management system should be established to ensure that all required documentation is recorded and maintained according to current standards and laws since the patient record is considered a legal document. As mentioned, practices should institute a documentation protocol to ensure that all providers are recording data in the same manner in order to decrease risk to the patient, practice, and provider. If any type of legal action is initiated, the dental record, which contains the details of patient care, is the vital document that can (or cannot) protect the oral healthcare provider. It is important to note that time and resources must be provided to train clinical personnel to properly utilize the practice management software program chosen by the practice. It is imperative that clinical personnel understand and know how to fully utilize the practice management software and how to document all required aspects of patient care in accordance with the practice's documentation protocol and standards of the profession.

The American Dental Hygienists' Association (ADHA) published the *Standards for Clinical Dental Hygiene Practice*, which provides a concise listing of documentation required at each phase of the dental hygiene process of care: assessment, dental hygiene diagnosis, planning, implementation, and evaluation (ADPIE).[14] These standards can be used when creating the documentation protocol specific to dental hygiene care. Once created, the protocol can be converted into a quality assurance audit: a quality assurance checklist to assess the overall effectiveness of each dental hygiene provider in relation to documentation within the patient record. For example, the standards itemize the required components of a comprehensive clinical assessment to be completed by the dental hygienist. As stated in the standards, "[C]omponents of the clinical assessment include an examination of the head and neck and oral cavity including an oral cancer screening, documentation of normal or abnormal findings, and assessment of the temporomandibular function. A current, complete set of radiographs provides needed data for a comprehensive dental and periodontal assessment". A comprehensive periodontal examination and hard-tissue evaluation that includes charting of existing conditions and habits and necessary radiographs and intraoral photographs are also part of the clinical assessment.[14] Criteria for the periodontal examination and hard-tissue evaluation are succinctly defined. Box 1.4 illustrates the criteria for a comprehensive periodontal examination.

In 2011, the American Academy of Periodontology (AAP) published a statement that is in agreement with the ADHA criteria, including that patients should receive a comprehensive periodontal evaluation annually, at a minimum, and more frequently if the patient's status dictates.[16] Therefore, a practices documentation protocol for a periodontal examination during the assessment phase of care should include the ADHA

• BOX 1.4   ADHA Standards of Clinical Dental Hygiene Practice

Comprehensive Periodontal Examination Assessment Criteria

A comprehensive periodontal examination is part of clinical assessment. It includes the following:

A. Full-mouth periodontal charting, including the following data points reported by location, severity, quality, written description, or numerically:
  1. Probing depths
  2. Bleeding points
  3. Suppuration
  4. Mucogingival relationships/defects
  5. Recession
  6. Attachment level/attachment loss
B. Presence, degree, and distribution of plaque and calculus
C. Gingival health/disease
D. Bone height/bone loss
E. Mobility and fremitus
F. Presence, location, and extent of furcation involvement

---

components and should be updated annually as per the AAP statement.

A quality assurance audit schedule should be established for the patient record. These "chart audits" must be formalized, objective, and completed to verify compliance with the documentation protocol, to ensure that the treatment delivered to patients meets the standards of care, and to protect the practice and providers from potential litigation.

The process domain of quality assessment includes the technical skills of the provider. A dental practice must apply the quality assurance mindset and verify the skills of all clinical personnel upon hire and periodically thereafter. In research, this process would be referred to as interexaminer reliability. Simply stated, this is a determination of the consistency of assessment findings among multiple (more than one) examiners. This quality assurance audit would include visual observations and outcome verification of findings to determine consistency among providers.

Documentation and communication within the outcomes domain include patient satisfaction surveys. Ultimately, if a patient is not satisfied with the overall experience with practice and the outcomes of care, they will find another dental practice. Patient satisfaction surveys should assess all aspects of the patient experience, including the facility itself, interactions and communication with personnel in administrative and clinical positions, and perceptions of clinical care received. These assessments are subjective but can provide valuable feedback regarding how the practice is viewed from a patient perspective.

Communication

Communication is defined as a process by which information is exchanged between and among individuals using a common system of signs, symbols, or behaviors.[3] We communicate in four basic ways, although there is often overlap and interaction among them: verbal, nonverbal, visual, and written. *Verbal* communication can be conducted face-to-face, via the telephone, or by using electronic conferencing. *Nonverbal* communication can involve facial expressions, gestures, eye contact, posture, body movements, and touch. Examples of *visual* communication include presentations, images, demonstrations, videos, and that may be misinterpreted are equally important. Dental hygienists should never provide treatment for which they are not qualified, educated, experienced, or licensed to perform.

Dental hygienists should carry adequate professional liability insurance and be familiar with the policy and its coverage, terms, and requirements. Understanding the nature of the coverage provided by a policy is essential. Claims-made coverage is limited to protection for allegations that arise from treatment rendered and reported while the policy is in force. Policy terms to consider include liability limits and deductibles. The types of insurance available and requirement for coverage can be different from state to state, and insurance policies must be carefully inspected so that the dental hygienist is fully aware of coverage and limitations. Many policies have restrictions or mandates for reporting if and when the hygienist is faced with a potential lawsuit. It also is advisable to contact an attorney for advice before entering into any binding agreement or when confronted with situations that have legal implications.

Social Media

The various types of electronic communications that are used in today's world have benefits and risks in both personal and professional settings. Blogs, microblogs, social networking, and media sharing are all considered types of **social media**.[20] These tools can be used for networking, promoting oral health, and increasing knowledge about oral health approaches and products as well as for everyday communications.

The same ethical and legal standards and practices applied in dental clinical settings should be adhered to when utilizing social media. The gift of trust that patients extend to their oral healthcare professionals must be treated with the utmost care. Confidentiality of patient information must be maintained and any breach of privacy could result in civil and criminal penalties. Every digital action, including a visit to a website, leaves a digital footprint that cannot be erased.[21] Keeping that fact uppermost in any electronic interaction will help in monitoring communication since publicly available content can reflect on an individual both personally and professionally. Numerous authors provide cautions that can guide the dental hygienist when utilizing social media[20–23]:

- Carefully view anything and everything that is posted online for its communication value and tone.
- Pause before posting. Strive to maintain personal and professional integrity at all times.
- Postings can be considered harassing or discriminatory in nature if they violate legal norms.
- Be vigilant about safeguarding health information privacy. Do not post any patient information.
- Do not give professional advice over social media platforms. You do not know the clinical circumstances, and doing so can be held against you.
- Do not "friend" or "like" patients on any social networking site. Keeping those boundaries is respectful and prudent.
- Know the rules and policies on social media of employers and related institutions.
- Do not post defamatory remarks about your employer, patients, colleagues, or other healthcare providers.
- Cyberbullying can occur either from peers or patients. Any bullying behavior should be reported and addressed.

Summary

The dental hygienist has the ability to consider and apply numerous strategies that can identify and reduce the risk of unwanted consequences that may occur in dental hygiene practice. Risk management and quality assurance practices, established as a system or individually, can enhance the health and safety of dental healthcare personnel and the dental patient and can support the ultimate goal of promoting oral health.

PRACTICE POINTER

As licensed dental health professionals, dental hygienists are legally and ethically required to adhere to the standards of care related to patient care. Licensed individuals are expected to be well versed regarding regulations governing their profession and to function within the state's practice act.

REFERENCES

1. Zarkowski P. Legal and ethical issues in the dental business office. In: Finkbeiner BL, Finkbeiner CA, eds. *Practice Management for the Dental Team*. 8th ed. Mosby; 2016:60–61.

2. Singh H. National Practitioner Data Bank. Generated using the Data Analysis Tool at https://www.npdb.hrsa.gov/analysistool. Data source: National Practitioner Data Bank (2021): Adverse Action and Medical Malpractice Reports (2011–March 31, 2021).

3. Donabedian A. Evaluating the quality of medical care. *Milbank Mem. Fund Q.* 1966;44(3):166–206. Reprinted in *Milbank Q.* 2005;83(4):691–729.

4. Health and Safety Executive (HSE). Risk Assessment Template 2019. https://www.hse.gov.uk/simple-health-safety/risk/risk-assessment-template-and-examples.htm. Accessed June 11, 2021.

5. American Health Information Management Association. Healthcare Documentation Quality Assessment and Management Best Practices. 2017. https://www.ahdionline.org/page/qa. Accessed July 2021.

6. Purtilo RB, Haddad AM, Doherty R. *Health Professional and Patient Interaction*. 8th ed. Saunders Elsevier; 2014.

7. United States Department of Labor, Occupational Safety and Health Administration (OSHA). Model Plans and Programs for the OSHA Bloodborne Pathogens and Hazard Communications Standards. https://www.osha.gov/sites/default/files/publications/osha3186.pdf. Accessed June 11, 2021.

8. United States Department of Labor, Occupational Safety and Health Administration (OSHA). Safety and Health Topics: Dentistry. https://www.osha.gov/dentistry. Accessed June 11, 2021.

9. United States Department of Health and Human Services. Health Information Privacy. https://www.hhs.gov/hipaa/index.html. Accessed June 11, 2021.

10. United States Department of Health and Human Services, Centers for Disease Control and Prevention (CDC). Infection Prevention Practices in Dental Settings: Basic Expectations for Safe Care. https://www.cdc.gov/oralhealth/infectioncontrol/summary-infection-prevention-practices/index.html. Accessed June 11, 2021.

11. United States Department of Health and Human Services, Centers for Disease Control and Prevention (CDC). Infection Prevention and Control in Dental Settings: Frequently Asked Questions. https://www.cdc.gov/oralhealth/infectioncontrol/faqs/index.html. Accessed July 13, 2021.

12. United States Department of Health and Human Services, Centers for Disease Control and Prevention (CDC). Infection Prevention Checklist for Dental Settings. https://www.cdc.gov/oralhealth/infectioncontrol/pdf/safe-care-checklist.pdf.

13. American Dental Association (ADA) and United States Department of Health and Human Services, US Public Health Service, US Food and Drug Administration (FDA). Dental Radiographic Examinations: Recommendations for Patient Selection and Limiting Radiation Exposure. 2012. https://www.fda.gov/media/84818/download. Accessed June 11, 2021.

14. American Dental Hygienists' Association (ADHA). Standards for Clinical Dental Hygiene Practice. 2016. https://www.adha.org/resources-docs/2016-Revised-Standards-for-Clinical-Dental-Hygiene-Practice.pdf.

15. Royal College of Dental Surgeons of Ontario. Dental Recordkeeping. 2019. https://az184419.vo.msecnd.net/rcdso/pdf/guidelines/RCDSO_Guidelines_Dental_Recordkeeping.pdf.

16. American Academy of Periodontology. Comprehensive periodontal therapy: a statement by the American Academy of Periodontology. *J Periodontol.* 2011;82:943–949.

17. American Dental Association. Glossary of Dental Administrative Terms. *Definition of Oral Health Literacy.* 2022. https://www.ada.org/publications/cdt/glossary-of-dental-administrative-terms.

18. American Psychological Association. APA Dictionary of Psychology. *Definition of Cultural Sensitivity.* 2022. https://dictionary.apa.org/cultural-sensitivity.

19. Institute of Medicine (IOM) and National Research Council (NRC). *Improving Access to Oral Health Care for Vulnerable and Underserved Populations.* The National Academies Press; 2011.

20. Sams LD. Understand the world of social media, *Dimens Dent Hyg.* 2013;11(12):57–63.

21. Oakley M, Spallek H. Social media in dental education: a call for research and action. *J Dent Educ.* 2012;76:279–287.

22. Henry RK. Maintaining professionalism in a digital age. *Dimens Dent Hyg.* 2012;10(10):28–32.

23. Carr MP. Lawsuit pending against Florida dental hygienist. *Dimens Dent Hyg.* 2018. https://dimensionsofdentalhygiene.com/lawsuit-pending-against-florida-dental-hygienist.

program, captures the essence of the public mission of the profession. The following, reprinted from Steele,[1] recalls that original oath, which has been updated since by the ADHA (http://www.adha.org/aboutadha/dhoath.htm):

> In my practice as a dental hygienist,
> I affirm my personal and professional commitment
> To improve the oral health of the public,
> To advance the art and science of dental hygiene,
> And to promote high standards of quality care.
> I pledge continually to improve my professional
> Knowledge and skills, to render a full measure
> Of service to each patient entrusted to my care,
> And to uphold the highest standards of professional
> Competence and personal conduct in the interest
> Of the dental hygiene profession and the public it serves.

Over the years, the profession of dental hygiene has evolved and changed with requirements for formalized education, regulation by licensure, and increased scope of practice. In addition, the public served by all healthcare providers has changed with the advent of new diseases, the development of advanced treatment methods, and a continually increasing human life span. However, dental hygiene retains its original focus on the public good, as well as its primary role in the prevention of dental disease and promotion of oral health.

Society recognizes that healthcare providers, by virtue of their education and special skills, are appropriately held to a higher standard than can be expressed exclusively by legislative mandate. Thus, these higher standards are expressed in professional codes of ethics and are enforced by those within the profession. This is called *self-regulating* or *self-policing behavior* and represents an increased level of trust on the part of the public. In essence, the public agrees that it is neither qualified nor in a position to evaluate the adequacy of treatment provided by healthcare professionals. Therefore, the public trusts these professionals to perform their own evaluations. Ethical dental hygienists willingly accept the **duty** of self-regulation, both in judging their colleagues and in submitting to **peer review,** to ensure quality care for the public.

The Healthcare Provider

All healthcare providers are granted special rights and responsibilities when they choose and enter a career in the biomedical field. In the past, becoming a professional in medicine, dentistry, or the allied disciplines was considered a calling. Once specialized training was completed, the individual became a member of a profession, defined as a limited group of persons who have acquired some special skill and are therefore able to perform that function in society better than the average person (Box 2.1).[2] In the corporate world, success is measured by financial gain. For the healthcare professional, the patient's welfare is placed above profit. Because of this ideal, society has granted the healthcare professional a certain status that carries prestige, power, and the right to apply specialized knowledge and skill.

When patients seek care from any healthcare provider, they expect to receive the best care from a professional and ethical practitioner. The healthcare services provided involve technical skill, appropriate knowledge, critical judgment, and—most importantly—caring. Patients perceive this essence of caring and respond to it. In the delivery of health care, trust is the critical foundation for the relationship that develops between the person seeking services—the patient or client—and the healthcare provider—the professional. The patient is aware that the healthcare provider has certain knowledge and skills; the graduation certificate and state license hanging on the wall are proof of that fact. However, the caring that the patient seeks gives the provider of dental hygiene services the greatest opportunity for professional service

---

• BOX 2.1   Characteristics of a True Profession

- Specialized body of knowledge of value to society
- Intensive academic course of study
- Standards of practice
- External recognition by society
- Code of ethics
- Organized association
- Service orientation

Data from: Motley WE. *Ethics, Jurisprudence and History for the Dental Hygienist.* 3rd ed. Lea & Febiger; 1983.

and satisfaction. An understanding of ethical issues and an awareness of the ethical obligations inherent in the provision of health care enable the dental hygienist to deal effectively with the problems of patients and their communities.

The importance and need for professionalism in all areas of health care have been extensively discussed and written about. Educators in medicine, dentistry, and dental hygiene have shared the importance of fostering professionalism and the fact that students must be immersed in clinical learning environments that model the highest principles.[3]

A number of medical organizations have focused on how to reemphasize the essence of professionalism in health care. The Institute of Medicine (now called the National Academy of Medicine) has produced several reports on this topic, and a project by a consortium of internal medicine groups led to the publication "Medical Professionalism in the New Millennium: A Physician Charter" (Physician Charter).[4] The authors advocated that everyone "involved in health care" use the charter to engage in discussions to strengthen the ethical underpinning of professional relationships. The Physician Charter sets out three fundamental principles that are not new but reinforce the foundation of the medical profession as one of service to others. The ethical principles of the primacy of patient welfare (beneficence and nonmaleficence) and patient autonomy are listed first; the principle of social justice is the third main tenet. The desired goal was to reinvigorate the value of professionalism that includes social responsibility: the ethic of care, and access to that care, for all members of society.

Professionalism is rooted in a relationship or contract with society. Ministry, medicine, and law grew from medieval guilds that were established in universities centuries ago. Entrance into these fields was controlled through the awarding of educational credentials. Early dental practitioners were itinerant barbers, and the road to professional status moved from apprenticeship to education through the establishment of professional schools.[5] Developing an educational process gave the members control over entry into the occupation and the size of the labor force. Because of their smaller number and their education, professionals became trustees of the community and took leadership positions in their societies.[6] This led to the public understanding that the professional person's

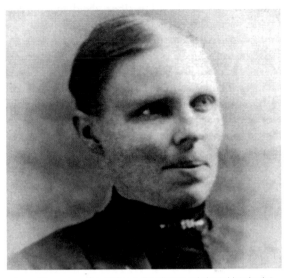

Irene Newman, the nation's first licensed dental hygienist.

knowledge is linked with service in the interest of the local community. Ultimately, the professional came to be defined as someone learned, publicly licensed, and supported by a collegial organization of peers committed to an ethic of service to clients and the public.[7] The professions then are much like universities and colleges in this sense—given a unique charter that grants autonomy and special status for a public purpose.

The Dental Hygienist

The dental hygienist is a professional oral healthcare provider—an individual who has completed a required higher-education accredited program; demonstrated knowledge, skills, and behaviors required by the college or university for graduation; passed a written national board examination; and successfully performed certain clinical skills on a state or regional examination. Because of these accomplishments, the state then grants this individual a license to practice the profession for which he or she completed training and education. By taking this step, the state is assuring the public that this licensed individual is competent to practice. That is the reason that a board of dentistry or a dental practice act exists: to protect the public's health and safety.

A dental hygienist provides educational, clinical, and therapeutic services supporting the total health of the patient through the promotion of optimal oral the types of professionals who are training together. The idea of training healthcare team members together has been met with great interest by students and faculty alike. Dental and dental hygiene educators have long acknowledged that oral health care is advanced when all members of the dental team are working together collaboratively. The preventive role of the dental hygienist is an excellent foundation for establishing oral and general community public health programs. Communicating with clinicians from all aspects of health care can only improve the outcomes for health, wellness, and treatment of diseases. Ethical issues will be encountered in interprofessional collaboration, and all members of healthcare teams will need to be aware of and trained in the complex dynamics of relationships.

Competency in Dental Hygiene

A basic attribute of professionals is that they have achieved **competency** in the scope of practice that is legally granted to that particular discipline or field. Competencies are the essential knowledge, skills, and abilities that are performed by a healthcare provider.[14] For a dental hygienist, competencies are skills regularly used in real practice settings to meet the oral health needs of patients. In addition, these competencies have been examined and endorsed by dental hygienists, dentists, and dental educators as valid and appropriate.

The Commission on Dental Accreditation, which is the authorized agency that accredits all dental hygiene education programs in the United States, publishes standards and competencies that all dental hygiene programs must meet or exceed in their educational programs (Box 2.2).

Accreditation in the United States is a system that has been developed to protect the public welfare and provide standards for the evaluation of educational programs and schools. Regional accrediting agencies examine colleges and universities, whereas specialized accrediting agencies focus on a particular profession or occupation. A specialized accrediting agency recognizes a course of instruction composed of a unique set of skills and knowledge, develops the accreditation standards by which such educational programs are evaluated, conducts evaluation of programs, and publishes a list of accredited programs that meet the national accreditation standards. Accreditation

standards are developed in consultation with those affected by the standards as well as those who represent the communities of interest.

The Commission on Dental Accreditation is the specialized accrediting agency recognized by the US Department of Education to **accredit** programs that provide basic preparation for licensure in dentistry, dental hygiene, and all related dental disciplines.[15] The commission consists of 30 members and includes a representative of the ADHA. The commission uses a peer-review process to ensure that the dental hygiene standards are met in each program, and a formal, on-site review is conducted every 7 years.

Patient care competencies, sometimes called *graduation competencies*, are standards that must be met by graduates of any educational program accredited by the Commission on Dental Accreditation. In states in which mastery of additional skills is mandated by the dental practice act, accredited programs also offer training opportunities in those competencies. An example of such a skill or function is the administration of local anesthesia or nitrous oxide analgesia.

Acquisition of dental hygiene skills is a process guided by educational theory and experienced dental hygiene educators. General education, biomedical science, dental science, and dental hygiene science content areas provide the core of knowledge in a dental hygiene program. Educational theory categorizes the process of skill performance into five stages of competency, also termed *the expert learning continuum* (Fig. 2.1). The five stages are novice, advanced beginner, competency, proficiency, and expertise.[16,17]

When a student begins preclinical activities and progresses to caring for clinical patients under the supervision of faculty, that stage of learning is called *novice* or *advanced beginner*. At or even before graduation, the student will have achieved competency—that is, the ability to perform skills without faculty supervision and with confidence. After graduation, the dental hygienist works toward proficiency and continues working, throughout his or her professional life, toward becoming an expert. Becoming an expert is not an endpoint; rather, it is something a true professional constantly strives for in practice. An analogy is a professional athlete who constantly practices a sport, seeking improvement and even greater ability. Perhaps that is why the term *practice* is used, as in the

> ### • BOX 2.2 Patient Care Competencies: Accreditation Standards for Dental Hygiene Education Programs
>
> The Commission on Dental Accreditation is the agency that conducts the accreditation program for all dental education programs. The Commission is the nationally recognized accrediting body for dentally related fields and receives its authority from acceptance by the dental community and by being recognized by the US Department of Education (USDE). The standards for dental hygiene are reviewed and revised periodically through an open and contributory process that includes representatives from the discipline of dental hygiene. The following standards may change because of this ongoing cycle of review but will include competencies in these areas:
>
> 1. Providing dental hygiene care for the child, adolescent, adult, geriatric, and special needs patient populations
> 2. Providing the dental hygiene process of care, which includes:
>   - Comprehensive collection of patient data to identify the patient's physical and oral health status
>   - Analysis of assessment findings and the use of critical thinking in order to address the patient's dental hygiene treatment needs
>   - Establishment of a dental hygiene care plan that reflects the realistic goals and treatment strategies to facilitate optimal oral health
>   - Provision of patient-centered treatment and evidence-based care in a manner minimizing risk and optimizing oral health
>   - Measurement of the extent to which goals identified in the dental hygiene care plan are achieved
>   - Complete and accurate recording of all documentation relevant to patient care
> 3. Providing dental hygiene care for all types of classifications periodontal disease, including patients who exhibit moderate to severe periodontal disease
> 4. Communicating and collaborating with other members of the healthcare team to support comprehensive patient care
> 5. Assessing, planning, implementing, and evaluating the health-promotion activities of community-based health-promotion and disease-prevention programs
> 6. Providing appropriate life-support measures for medical emergencies that may be encountered in dental hygiene practice
> 7. Applying the principles of ethical reasoning, ethical decision making, and professional responsibility as they pertain to the academic environment, research, patient care, and practice management
> 8. Applying legal and regulatory concepts to the provision and/or support of oral healthcare services
> 9. Applying self-assessment skills to prepare for lifelong learning
> 10. Evaluating current scientific literature
> 11. Problem-solving strategies related to comprehensive patient care and management of patients
>
> Data from: Commission on Dental Accreditation (CODA). *Accreditation Standards for Dental Hygiene Education Programs*. 2022. https://legacy.ada.org/en/coda/current-accreditation-standards.

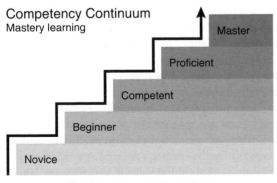

• **Fig. 2.1** Competency continuum.

practice of dental hygiene or the practice of dentistry. Professionals constantly seek to perform at increasingly higher levels, perfecting the art and science of dental hygiene for every patient treated.

Standards for Clinical Dental Hygiene Practice

The ADHA established **standards** for clinical dental hygiene practice in 1985 to outline the expectations for the practicing dental hygienist.[18] In its role as the that fosters an open exchange of information. Patients expect that personal, intimate facts and impressions about them will be kept in confidence by the dental hygienist.

Tolerance for Others

Treating all patients without discrimination is a basic ethical and legal requirement. This behavior goes beyond the legal warning to not discriminate based on race, creed, color, age, sex, ethnicity, or disabilities to include occupation, financial status, personality, and oral conditions. It means caring for all individuals who seek treatment whether or not they are likeable. Patients occasionally will prove difficult and hostile during the course of treatment, but dental hygienists must still treat such persons to the best of their ability.

Respect for Self

Dental hygienists should maintain their own physical and mental health so that the patient's needs can remain the primary focus. Working while under the influence of alcohol, drugs, lack of sleep, or emotional distress does not allow the healthcare provider to focus on the needs of the patient. Each patient deserves the complete attention of the dental hygienist while being treated.

Legal Requirements for the Dental Hygienist

Dental hygienists are subject to the rules and regulations of the jurisdiction in which they practice dental hygiene. When a license is granted to an individual, that person becomes responsible for knowing and upholding all the statutes and laws set down in the legal document, usually called the *state dental practice act* or the *code of dental practice*. Ignorance of a portion of the law or code is no excuse for noncompliance by a dental hygienist or any other healthcare provider. The responsibility and power for legislative protection of the public rest with each individual state or territory. **Licensure** is designed to enforce practice codes, establish standards, and sanction incompetent practitioners, all for the purpose of protecting the health and safety of the public.

The scope of practice of a dental hygienist was first established by law in Connecticut in 1915 at the urging of Dr. A. C. Fones, the father of dental hygiene.[2] The Connecticut dental law delineated the practice parameters of the dental hygienist and subsequently served as a model for the states that later adopted similar legislation. All state boards, as well as those in the Virgin Islands and Puerto Rico, grant a license to practice to the dental hygienist. An unlicensed person may not provide dental hygiene care.

Legal statutes periodically change in response to many factors, both to protect the public and advance the interests of the health professions. The process for any legal change is arduous, complicated, and costly in time and effort. Most legislative changes related to dental health care are driven by individuals in the dental and dental hygiene professions. For the most part, the public remains unaware of the intricacies of the process or its effect on the delivery of their dental healthcare. Some of the factors that influence legislative changes in a state include the following:

- Need and demand for dental care
- Distribution of dental healthcare providers
- Federal health legislation
- Goals of organized dental and dental hygiene associations advocacy groups

Increases in the scope of practice for the dental hygienist have occurred over the years but usually have been accompanied by a great deal of controversy and consternation. The services performed by the dental hygienist usually are classified as either traditional duties, such as scaling, root planing, and education of the patient, or expanded functions, such as the administration of local anesthesia and placement of restorative materials. Some states have implemented an additional practice level for dental hygienists, termed an *expanded-* or *extended-duty dental hygienist.* Individuals pursuing this level of practice must complete additional training in periodontal or restorative functions and must be sanctioned to perform these skills by the particular state in which they practice. The exact duties and services that may be performed by the dental hygienist in a particular state are based on customary parameters of practice, dental statutes, and the state dental practice act. Only duties or functions allowed in a particular state may be performed by the licensed dental hygienist, even if that individual is trained and licensed in another state where the practice act is more expansive.

The legal mandates in each state use terms that differentiate the level of supervision set out by that particular body. Some states are more liberal than others in their dental practice acts. Several states have adopted mechanisms to allow a dental hygienist to practice without the supervision of a dentist after gaining a special license or credential. These allowances are granted after additional training or testing, often with the goal of improving public access to appropriate care.

Summary

The profession of dental hygiene was established with the goal of providing oral health education and services to the public so that dental disease could be prevented. As a healthcare professional, the dental hygienist is given the trust of society, and with that special trust comes rights and responsibilities. Attaining and maintaining competency in dental hygiene are among the obligations that the dental hygienist accepts in completing a formal education program and passing the state licensure examination. The traits that characterize a successful dental hygienist are the same traits found in any successful healthcare professional: placing the needs of the patient first and aiming to provide the best care to every patient as well as society at large.

REFERENCES

1. Steele PF. *Dimensions of Dental Hygiene*. 3rd ed. Lea & Febiger; 1983:477.
2. Motley WE. *Ethics, Jurisprudence and History for the Dental Hygienist*. 3rd ed. Lea & Febiger; 1983.
3. Beemsterboer PL. Developing an ethic of access to care in dentistry. *J Dent Educ*. 2006;70(11):1212.
4. ABIM Foundation; ACP-ASIM Foundation; European Federation of Internal Medicine. Medical professionalism in the new millennium: a physician charter. *Ann Intern Med*. 2002;136(3):243–246.
5. Ring ME. *Dentistry: An Illustrated History*. Abrams; 1992.
6. Brint S. *In an Age of Experts: The Changing Role of Professionals in Politics and Public Life*. Princeton University Press; 1994.
7. Sullivan WM. *Work and Integrity*. 2nd ed. Jossey-Bass; 2005.
8. Stern DT. *Measuring Medical Professionalism*. Oxford University Press; 2006.
9. Ozar DT. Three models of professionalism and professional obligation in dentistry. *J Am Dent Assoc*. 1985;110:173.
10. Institute of Medicine (IOM). *Crossing the Quality Chasm*. National Academy Press; 2001.
11. Institute of Medicine (IOM). *Health Professions Education: A Bridge to Quality*. National Academy Press; 2003.
12. Formicola AJ, Andrieu SC, Buchanan JA, Childs GS, Gibbs M, Inglehart MR, Kalenderan E, Pyle MA, D'Abreu K, Evans L. Interprofessional education in U.S. and Canadian dental schools: an ADEA team study group report. *J Dent Educ*. 2012;76(9):1250–1268.
13. Interprofessional Education Collaborative Expert Panel. *Core Competencies for Interprofessional Collaborative Practice: Report of an Expert Panel*. Interprofessional Education Collaborative. 2011. https://www.aacom.org/docs/default-source/insideome/ccrpt05-10-11.pdf.
14. Beemsterboer PL. Competency in allied dental education. *J Dent Educ*. 1994;11:19.
15. Commission on Dental Accreditation (CODA). Accreditation Standards for Dental Hygiene Education Programs. 2022. https://legacy.ada.org/en/coda/current-accreditation-standards.
16. Chambers DW. Toward a competency-based curriculum. *J Dent Educ*. 1993;57:790.
17. Chi MT, Glaser R, Farr M, *The Nature of Expertise*. Lawrence Erlbaum; 1988.
18. American Dental Hygienists' Association. Standards for Clinical Dental Hygiene Practice. 2016. https://www.adha.org/resources-docs/2016-Revised-Standards-for-Clinical-Dental-Hygiene-Practice.pdf.

as well. That is why differentiating right from wrong, which is a cognitive matter, is different from incorporating right and wrong into life—that is, into moral development overall. The examples of saints and heroes, including highly admirable members of one's own profession, as well as moral growth by ordinary people every day, can give clues about the causes or mechanisms of moral development. Since psychological research on moral development is a fairly new field, from a scientific point of view much of what is involved remains unclear.

What has become clear is that a strong relationship exists between education and the development of moral judgment, which is the cognitive aspect of moral development. One of the strongest and most consistent correlates with the development of moral judgment, even stronger than chronologic age, is years of formal education.[1,2] For many people, moral development continues as long as the person is in a formal education environment, but then it plateaus upon leaving school. This provides an important lesson: If you want to keep growing as a moral human being, keep learning, though not necessarily in school. Instead, never stop observing and reflecting on what is going on around you and people's reasons for their actions. Keep asking questions, read and discuss with others to keep your learning vital, and above all do so in aspects of your life in which moral matters are at stake. Professional life obviously is one of those aspects.

Various educational programs and interventions have been used to facilitate the development of moral judgment by providing enriched and stimulating educational experiences. A review of moral education programs revealed that almost half were effective in promoting moral development, especially if the program lasted longer than a few weeks and involved the participants in discussions of controversial moral dilemmas.[3] Adults also seemed to gain more from such programs than did younger children, most likely because a wider range of life experiences typically enriches a person's awareness of the moral aspects of situations.

These findings have implications for persons preparing for a career in dental hygiene because they emphasize several things about learning to make moral decisions. First, findings suggest that the capacity for moral judgment is not as rigid as some have argued—that is, neither a person's cognitive moral development nor their ability to employ what they understand in actual decisions is frozen at some specified age. Rather, individuals can continue to learn, and research has supported the idea that adults make greater gains than children. Second, individuals who are still in formal education programs will likely benefit from advanced training, especially when expected to exercise their ethical decision-making ability by considering a variety of dental hygiene case scenarios. Third, these findings suggest that participation in continuing education courses after graduation may reinforce an individual's ability to make sound ethical judgments and also have a positive impact on the person's commitment to practicing in an ethical manner.

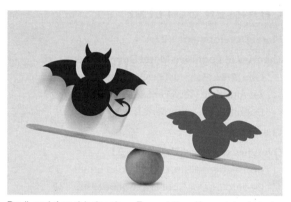

Devil and Angel balancing. From: https://www.istockphoto.com.

Theories of Cognitive Moral Development

One View: Male Justice Orientation

Psychologists have done some of the most important work in developing our knowledge about moral development and how it influences our actions in adulthood. Two of the most famous developmental psychologists, Piaget[4] and Kohlberg,[5] categorized stages in the moral development of male children. Piaget and Kohlberg both stated that moral development is sequential and depends on an individual's level of cognitive development. Piaget's[4] model consisted of four stages (Table 3.1), whereas Kohlberg[5] defined moral development according to both levels and stages (Table 3.2).

Each stage in the process of cognitive moral development involves judgment skills that are more

TABLE 3.1	Piaget's Four-Stage Model of Moral Development	
Stage	**Characteristics of Moral Development**	
1	Amoral stage (ages 0 to 2 years)	
2	Egocentric stage (ages 2 to 7 years); bends rules and reacts to environment instinctively	
3	Heteronomous stage (ages 7 to 12 years); accepts the moral authority of others	
4	Autonomous stage (ages 12 and older); a morality of self based on cooperation; rules tested and become internalized	

complex, comprehensive, and differentiated from the preceding stage. The process also is sequential, with an individual moving from simple to more complex stages. Kohlberg's stages follow the Piagetian view that justice is the core of morality; however, because this was first demonstrated empirically only in male subjects, it is important not to generalize more broadly at this point. Kohlberg's theory focuses primarily on cognitive processes, which is consistent with his belief that understanding guides behavior. He asserts the moral superiority of his stage 6, where what he considers to be genuine moral judgments are made and where genuine moral judgments are defined as judgments about the good and right of actions based on

objective, impersonal, or ideal grounds.[6] Thus, cognitive moral development for Kohlberg is a progression toward increasingly valid or universal moral thought. There are other accounts of genuine moral judgments besides Kohlberg's, however, so the healthcare provider should consider what more there is to cognitive moral development than Kohlberg has discussed and what else besides the cognitive aspects goes into moral development more broadly.

An Alternate View: Female Ethic of Care

Among the criticisms of Kohlberg's work is the challenge that his model reflects a male-oriented perspective of morality. Gilligan,[7] in her classic book *In a Different Voice*, states that women tend to see morality in the context of a relationship she calls the *ethic of care*. She proposes that feminine **moral reasoning** is typically different from masculine moral reasoning. To survive evolutionarily and practically, female individuals have had to develop a sense of responsibility based on the universal principle of caring, which Gilligan sees as quite different from universal justice. Like Kohlberg's model, Gilligan's model also has three levels (Table 3.3); unlike Kohlberg's model, Gilligan includes noncognitive growth in her model of moral development.

Gilligan believes that complete moral development occurs in the context of two moral orientations—a male justice orientation and a female ethic of care—and, therefore, that Kohlberg's measurement of moral development *only* in a justice-oriented scoring system

TABLE 3.2	Kohlberg's Three-Level Model of Moral Development	
Level	**Level of Reasoning**	**Stage**
1	Preconventional reasoning (stages 1 and 2), in which externally established rules determine right and wrong action	Stage 1: punishment and obedience orientation Stage 2: instrumental relativist orientation
2	Conventional reasoning (stages 3 and 4), in which expectations of family and groups are maintained and where loyalty and conformity are considered important	Stage 3: interpersonal concordance orientation Stage 4: law and order orientation
3	Postconventional or principled (stages 5 and 6), in which the person autonomously examines and defines moral values with decisions of conscience dictating the right action	Stage 5: social contract legalistic orientation Stage 6: universal ethical principle orientation

this action would be enhanced oral health for the patient. However, in some states removal of overhangs may be illegal for a hygienist, and doing so could put a professional reputation in jeopardy or make employer communication difficult. Third, the hygienist could discuss with the employer the fact that overhangs are frequently present. The consequences could be that the dentist would restore teeth more carefully. However, another consequence might be that the dentist simply tells the hygienist to just do her job. If the hygienist persists, the employer may decide to terminate employment. All these are consequences to consider because they are important alternatives for the dental hygienist in this situation. However, notice that the consequential reasoning approach would require the hygienist to do what is the best action for good even when it might not be in the hygienist's own best interest. Being ethical is not always easy, and most versions of consequentialism stress that in good moral reasoning the effects of the alternative actions for everyone affected, not just oneself, must be taken into account.

John Stuart Mill was one of the most famous proponents of **utilitarianism,** a version of the consequentialist approach to moral decision making, who stressed that in consequentialist reasoning, every person affected by an action should be considered.[11] Mill often is described as saying that an action should be judged to be moral on its capacity to provide the greatest good for the largest number of people. However, his teacher Bentham said that, not Mill, and Bentham himself eventually repudiated the phrase because it misled people into thinking that, for a utilitarian, whatever benefitted the *majority* was the right thing to do. Both men did teach that the moral action is the one (of the alternative actions available) that maximizes good and minimizes harm when the consequences for every affected person are considered. Obviously, one place where utilitarian reasoning might be appropriate is when ethical matters must be decided (e.g., by a legislator or officer of government) that affect large social systems, a community, or even a nation. A public health dentist or a hygienist with a master's degree in public health would be more likely to use this approach in public health thinking than would others. Thus, one of the best examples of utilitarianism in dentistry is the application of fluoride to community water systems. The consequence was a benefit through caries reduction, provided at a relatively low cost, and available to all members of a community regardless of social status or income, and with almost no possibility of causing harm. The alternative, going on without fluoride, was a situation in which many people would have had many more carious lesions and other dental problems because their oral hygiene was typically not dependable enough to prevent these harms.

Deontology, or Nonconsequentialism

NONCONSEQUENTIALIST ETHICS

An action is right when it conforms to a principle or rule of conduct that meets a requirement of some overriding duty.

The expression *deontological ethics* is derived from the Greek word *deon,* meaning "duty." Deontologists state that some actions are required by the rightness or wrongness of the action, regardless of the consequences of the action. Whereas consequentialists focus on the consequences of an act, deontologists argue that some acts are right or wrong independent of their consequences (thus the term **nonconsequentialism**). Some acts are right because they have a direct relation to some overriding duty, or they are wrong because they directly violate some overriding duty, but not because of consequences. For example, a deontologist might believe that a healthcare provider, as a moral person, has a duty to tell the truth in all circumstances and therefore has a specific duty to tell the truth to patients. With this view, a professional's duty to tell the truth to a patient is not founded on the consequences of telling the patient the truth, but on the belief either that an absolute duty exists never to lie or that the patient is entitled by reason of a fundamental right to receive the truth. According to deontology, then, moral standards exist independently of the particular circumstances of an action and do not depend on consequences. Duty and the relation of a person's actions to duty are the only relevant considerations.

Immanuel Kant[12] is credited for establishing one of the most detailed nonconsequentialist or deontological theories of ethical thinking. Kant held that the test of any rule of conduct is whether it can be a duty for all human beings to act on—what he called a *universal law.* That test is, for Kant, what tells us whether an action is directly related to an overriding duty. Kant also stressed that all human beings (as adults) are free, are worthy of respect, and are their own choosers of their purposes and actions. Many deontological theories of human rights have been built by later thinkers on this basis.[12] This school of thought has had a significant effect on biomedical ethics. It places primacy on the right of the individual to act autonomously—that is, to make his or her own decisions on the basis of his or her own values, goals, principles, and ideals. Autonomy as an important principle of healthcare ethics is further explored in Chapter 4.

Kant's test for correct moral reasoning was called *the categorical imperative,* which means a rule or standard of conduct that is absolutely binding for all human beings under all circumstances in which the rule or standard applies. Kant held that some of the moral rules we are familiar with (e.g., Do not lie) have this character of overriding duty. Most of the rules with this character are negative, in that they tell a person what *not* to do—for example, one must not lie, cheat, or steal. Borrowing an old Latin word, *perfectum,* which means "binding unconditionally," Kant categorized the negative rules having this character as "perfect duties." Perfect duties are always binding. Kant also talked about "imperfect duties," which refer to moral obligations to act in certain ways during our lives but leave it to each person to judge when and in what situation to fulfill the obligation (*imperfect* here meaning "conditionally binding"—that is, depending on the actor's judgment to determine when to fulfill the obligation). Thus, a perfect duty requires one not to kill an innocent human being. The prohibition against murder is binding because it is right and directly connected to an overriding duty, not because of the consequences. An example of an imperfect duty is an obligation to help another person in need or to be compassionate. We all have an overriding duty to pay attention to people's needs, but we are not obligated to try to meet them in every situation in which someone is in need. It is a matter of moral judgment that a person must carefully make to determine for whom and in which situations to fulfill this duty.[12]

Sometimes Kant's categorical imperative is compared with the golden rule, which cautions individuals to "Do unto others as you would have others do unto you." As Kant stated it, "Act that you can will the maxim of your action to be a universal law binding upon the will of every other rationale person."[12]

An example of the deontological approach as it applies to dental hygiene is that a hygienist has a duty to maintain patient confidentiality in the provision of oral health care for his or her patient. Other than sharing information appropriately with other healthcare providers, information acquired while providing patient care must remain private unless the patient's express permission has been granted. If an adult patient's relative or a representative of a finance company asks questions regarding the patient, for example, confidentiality must be maintained. It is right because respect for others' autonomy is an overriding duty, and a patient's revelation of personal information to the hygienist for purposes of oral health care does not include permission to use it for any other purpose. If this philosophy were strictly held in health care, public health reporting of communicable diseases would seem to not be permitted. However, Kant expanded his moral theory to cover societal rules in ways that could make such reporting morally acceptable if one could reasonably argue that any rational person would want such information communicated to avoid harm to others. Just as consequentialist thinking can get quite complex when many alternative actions must be compared, when consequences are hard to predict, and when different kinds of benefits and harms affect different persons as a consequence of an action, so deontological thinking—though it may appear simple at the start—can be complex when trying to determine what social standards could reasonably be willed by rational people to be universal standards to live by. No moral philosopher has ever claimed that moral thinking is like solving a simple equation in mathematics. One reason theories have been offered is to help us understand how complex making good moral decisions can be, and then to try to help us think about them more clearly.

Virtue Ethics

VIRTUE ETHICS

Character or virtue and the goodness of the person in living a good life is acquired by a person through learning and reflection and repetition (based on the Greek traditions of Plato and Aristotle).

4

Ethical Principles and Values

KRISTIN MINIHAN-ANDERSON

CHAPTER OUTLINE

LEARNING OUTCOMES

- Identify the four fundamental ethical principles.
- Define the terms *autonomy, confidentiality, societal trust, nonmaleficence, beneficence, justice,* and *fidelity.*
- Describe the difference between a choice and an ethical dilemma.
- Explain the role of principles in the decision-making process of the dental hygienist.
- Identify the components of informed consent.
- Discuss the three types of informed consent.
- Compare the values and ethical concepts that support the principles of ethics.

Ethical principles guide the conduct of healthcare providers by helping to identify, clarify, and justify moral choices. Principles help address this moral question: What should I do in the situation I now face? More specifically, what is good, right, or proper for a person to do in this situation? Normative ethics seeks to classify actions as either right or wrong and provide a set of norms for action by developing rules that govern human conduct. Normative principles provide a cognitive framework for analyzing moral questions and problems. These principles are linked to commonly expected behaviors because they are based on shared standards of thinking and behaving. In health care, the main normative principles are nonmaleficence, beneficence, autonomy, and justice. These principles are associated with expectations for behavior, and they provide guidelines for dealing with right and wrong actions. These principles provide direction about what should and should not be done in specific situations.

Ethical Dilemmas

A difference exists between addressing everyday problems and addressing ethical dilemmas. An ethical

Application of Beneficence

For dental hygienists, whose primary focus is preventing oral diseases, promoting good is a daily purpose and goal. Indeed, for any person who is in a position to promote good for the benefit of others, as healthcare providers are, failure to increase the good of others is morally wrong. The purpose and existence of biomedical research, public health policies and programs, and preventive medicine are the formalized aspects of this part of health care. Through various federal, state, and community-based activities, society attempts to meet this need for the good of the public. The promotion of good becomes difficult, however, when good is defined according to differing values and belief systems. The teaching of careful oral hygiene self-care to maintain health and function is an example of promotion of good to many people. However, the removal of all carious teeth to eliminate pain and suffering may be considered promoting good to other individuals. In public health programs, the appropriation of limited resources to meet the medical and dental needs of a given population can be a challenging and frustrating exercise but also part of being a healthcare professional who advocates for the betterment of society.

Principle of Autonomy

Autonomy is self-determination and the ability to be self-governing and self-directing. An autonomous person chooses thoughts and actions relevant to his or her needs, independent from the will of others. In health care, autonomy gives rise to the concept of permitting individuals to make decisions about their own health, which is the heart of many ethical dilemmas that occur in dentistry.[6] When weighed against competing principles, autonomy may be overridden. It also does not extend to persons who lack the capacity to act autonomously, such as children and those with certain intellectual and developmental disabilities (IDDs), neurological disabilities, or mental illnesses.[7] All healthcare providers must respect the autonomy of patients and properly inform them about all aspects of the diagnosis, prognosis, and care being provided. Because dental hygienists have a wide range of knowledge and skills, they must fully and adequately explain the parameters of the services that can be performed, as well as the consequences of performing or not performing those services.

Application of Autonomy

The application of autonomy is founded in deontology and is based on respect for persons. Essentially, deontology expounds that lying is always wrong because if everyone lied then human communications would break down entirely.[3] The deontologist holds that the healthcare provider has a duty to allow patients to make decisions about actions that will affect their bodies. The healthcare provider also has a duty to provide patients with all the unbiased information they would need to make a decision about treatment options. This is an area in which potential for conflict exists between what the provider believes is in the best interest of the patient and what the patient believes is in his or her best interest. Sometimes what the provider believes is best for the patient is not what the patient elects to do. As long as the patient selects treatment options that are consistent with accepted standards of care, the professional may ethically act on the patient's choice. However, the professional practitioner also has the autonomy to not provide a service requested by the patient if that service is in conflict with the standards of patient care. Referring back to the ethical dilemma presented earlier in this chapter, refusing a patient's request to proceed with crown and root debridement without him taking the required antibiotic premedication would be ethical even though that decision would conflict with the patient's autonomy. Dentists and hygienists must avoid doing harm to a patient even if the patient is exercising autonomy by asking to receive a potentially harmful treatment or service. The provider's obligation to adhere to the principles of nonmaleficence and beneficence overrides the patient's right to autonomy. Additionally, refusing a patient's request to provide services not aligned with the standards of care protects the provider from possible liability and litigation should harm come to the patient.

Principle of Justice

The principle of **justice** is generally interpreted as fair, equitable, and appropriate treatment of persons.[7] Non-consequentialists view justice as a duty for healthcare providers. The most fundamental principle of justice was defined by the Greek philosopher Aristotle: Equals should be treated equally and unequals unequally.[8] This means that individuals should be treated the same unless the ways in which they differ is relevant to the situation at hand. For example, if a man and woman are doing the same job and no relevant differences exist between the work they perform and deliver, then it is *just* to pay them the same wages. If the man is paid more than the woman simply because he is a man, this is *unjust* as it constitutes discrimination.[8] Providing special treatment based upon race, sex, age, religious beliefs, or socioeconomic status is considered unjust.

There are many categories of justice, and the one most applicable to bioethics and most often discussed in terms of public policy issues is referred to as *distributive justice.* It is believed by many ethicists that the conflicts of interest that arise when resources are scarce, and differing opinions exist as to how those resources should be allocated have created the need for society to have reasonable policies to determine what people deserve.[8] Resources can include facilities, materials, specially trained individuals, money, or time. **Distributive justice** is concerned with the fair and equitable delivery of healthcare resources determined by societal norms that support social cooperation.[7] Policymakers must confront the issue of how society distributes its resources. Various principles of distributive justice can be applied alone or in combination to form balanced decisions, and some are deemed justifiable and socially acceptable criteria for not treating people the same. The following are some valid principles with examples for distribution to each person[7]:

- An equal share: Following a natural disaster, everyone in the community is provided the same quantity of bottles of drinking water.
- According to need: The government provides benefits to those who are in need according to the Federal Poverty Guidelines. If the inclusion criteria are not met, then no benefits are provided.
- According to effort: The person who wakes up early to be first in line for tickets to a baseball game between their favorite team and the team's rival gets first choice of the best seats.
- According to merit: Only those who contribute the most to improving an organization receive a promotion and pay raise.

Application of Justice

If resources were unlimited, the problem of just allocation would be minimal. Unfortunately, that is not the reality of the world in which we live. Choices must be made, benefits and burdens must be balanced, and resources must be justly distributed. A lofty goal for most organized societies would be the just application of health care. However, no legal mandate exists for free medical and dental care to be available to all persons, and decisions are made daily according to the ability of the patient to pay for the services rendered. This means the provision of dental care is applied unequally. People who present for treatment are, for the most part, granted access to care based on their economic ability and not their dental needs. This creates access to care issues.

The question of who should provide dental care when an individual of low socioeconomic status (SES) is in need of treatment is difficult to answer. Many dental hygienists and dentists provide charitable services on a regular basis, either in a private practice office or through participation in a community-based service event, because of their recognition of their obligation to serve society. Unfortunately, although this is a lauded practice, it does not come close to meeting the needs of those who cannot access dental care. Many dental public health practitioners and leaders consistently advocate for the profession to make oral health a much higher priority for federal and state decision makers.

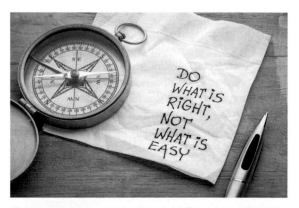

"Do what is right, not what is easy." From: https://www.istockphoto.com.

decision-making capacity to consent to treatment and is seeking treatment voluntarily, meaning of her or his own free will and not being subjected to coercion.

Informed consent is two pronged. First, the information component involves discussion and full disclosure of all relevant information needed to make a decision. This discussion should use language that is easy to understand and discloses to the patient the diagnosis, description, and purpose of the treatment planned, benefits and risks of proposed treatment, alternative treatment options, prognosis of no treatment, costs, and time frame of treatment, and it should specify the provider of care. Second, during the consent component, the patient makes a decision on the basis of the information provided and authorizes the clinician to proceed.

Several criteria are involved in informed consent, and it is an ongoing process, meaning that the discussion between provider and patient continues throughout the length of treatment. The patient is informed of progress, lack of progress, and treatment goals met. If any aspect of the treatment agreed upon is going to be changed, the patient must be informed of the changes and provide consent to those changes.

Application of Informed Consent

As previously noted in the discussion of autonomy, accepting the decision of the patient when it is in conflict with what the healthcare provider would most likely recommend is extremely difficult for dental professionals. Dentists and dental hygienists must recognize that the patient has a right to informed consent as well as a right to make an informed refusal. Autonomy includes the right for a patient to assess all the information provided by the professional regarding the proposed treatment and to refuse the recommendations in part or whole. This is known as *informed refusal*. From a risk management standpoint, it is imperative to have an office policy to ensure that the informed consent process is carried out for all patients and to obtain a signed refusal-of-treatment form if a patient declines the recommended treatment.[11,12] As discussed in Chapter 1, the principle of autonomy cannot supersede the provider's obedience to the standards of care. If the patient's refusal requires the clinician to deviate from the standards of care, the clinician would risk

exposure to liability as that deviation could constitute negligence and/or malpractice. When a patient's values and expectations are in conflict with a clinician's legal and ethical duties, the provider must consider dismissing the patient from the practice. Discontinuation of the provider–patient relationship is discussed in Chapter 9.

Patients provide their authorization for a comprehensive treatment plan when they grant the healthcare provider informed consent for that treatment. There are basically three types of informed consent:

1. Implied consent: Consent is not formal. Patient passively cooperates without extensive discussion and is given simply enough information for a process or procedure to be understood. This type of consent is considered adequate for the assessment, diagnosis, and planning components of the dental hygiene process of care.
2. Verbal consent: Consent in which the patient verbally consents to a process or procedure but does not provide a signature on a form. Diagnostic procedures such as exposing radiographs and routine prophylaxis, use of medicaments such as topical anesthetic, noninjectable anesthetic, dentinal desensitizers, and various forms of fluoride are considered acceptable with verbal consent. These procedures are documented in the patient record but do not typically require a patient signature.
3. Written consent: This type of consent is necessary for any procedures or treatments beyond those listed above. Use of anesthesia, debridement beyond prophylaxis, and invasive, irreversible procedures, and surgical procedures would require written consent with a patient signature.

Not all individuals have the ability to make informed decisions about their dental health. Children, people who have intellectual and developmental disabilities, neurologic disabilities, or mental illness typically have a parent or legal guardian who assumes that function. Depending on the age and capacity of the child, certain choices can and should be discussed with the younger patient, but actual decisions regarding what types of services are rendered must remain the purview of the legal guardian. When the patient does not understand because of a language barrier, informed consent is not possible, and steps must be taken to remedy the situation. The use of a translator, family member, or other communication option must be pursued to ensure that the patient fully understands the choices and consequences. To do any less is unethical and illegal. The only exception to this would be an emergency when delayed treatment could put the patient's life in danger and an immediate procedure is required to save that life.

Capacity

When discussing the topic of decision-making from a bioethical standpoint, **capacity** is the ability of a patient to understand the benefits and risks of, and the alternatives to, a proposed treatment or intervention, including no treatment.[13] The terms *capacity* and *competency* are often used interchangeably; however, there is a difference in how each is determined. Capacity is determined by a healthcare provider regarding an individual's ability to make an informed decision. Competency speaks to one's ability to participate in legal proceedings and is determined in the courts by a judge. When evaluating capacity, four key components are usually assessed: (1) *understanding* the situation, (2) *appreciating* the consequences of one's decision, (3) *reasoning* and rationalization in one's thought process, and (4) ability to *communicate* one's choices and wishes. A patient's capacity is assessed informally during all encounters but may need to be assessed formally if there is an acute change in cognition and/or mental status. For an individual to give informed consent, capacity is a prerequisite. This is a growing concern with an aging population as older adults can exhibit a wide range of cognitive function and neurologic disabilities. Older individuals are not only becoming a larger percentage of the population, but they are also living longer. The US Census Bureau predicts that one of every five Americans will be 65 years of age or older by the year 2030.[14]

Providers may also need to assess the capacity of a patient who may be under the influence of substances such as illicit as well as legally obtained alcohol and drugs. Use and misuse of substances can affect the central nervous system and distort one's perceptions of situations and the environment due to the physiologic impact of these substances. Following the ADHA's health history criteria outlined in the Standards of Clinical Dental Hygiene Practice can help identify potential issues related to substance use and misuse. These criteria include the assessment of demographic information, vital signs, physical characteristics, social history, medical history, and pharmacologic history. It is imperative for providers to engage in meaningful continuing education regarding the recognition and management of patients who may be misusing substances to ensure that they are not exposed to undo liability.

Questioning the patient as to how he or she understands the risks of treatment or why they are declining treatment are among the ways to explore the capacity of a patient. Objective assessment instruments can be utilized to help with this determination and are routinely used by primary healthcare providers.[15] Treating a person with a cognitive impairment can present a range of ethical dilemmas.

In the dental setting, ensuring that a patient has capacity may often require reaching out to the family, primary care physician, or surrogate decision maker. It is not uncommon for an individual to have transient or diminished capacity, which is the ability to express his or her wishes on one day and not the next. Awareness of the issues of capacity will assist the dental hygienist in providing ethical and legal oral health treatment to geriatric, and all, populations.

Confidentiality

Confidentiality is a critical aspect of trust in the provider–patient relationship and has a long history of use in health care. Confidentiality is related to the obligation a provider has to keep safe a patient's protected health information (PHI) unless consent has been provided by the patient to release information in a controlled manner. The patient has a reasonable expectation that PHI will be kept private. The requirement for confidentiality is mentioned in all codes of ethics as well as in the Hippocratic Oath. Trust is necessary for the exchange of personal and intimate information from the patient to the clinician. A patient has a right to privacy concerning his or her medical and dental history, examination findings, discussion of treatment options and treatment choices, and all records pertaining to dental and dental hygiene care. This privacy extends to the way in which information is gathered, stored, and communicated to other healthcare professionals. Discussion about a patient's history or treatment is not to be shared with spouses, family, or friends—to do so is a violation of confidentiality. Legal requirements regarding the confidentiality of PHI are discussed in Chapter 1. Information about a patient can be given to other healthcare professionals with the patient's permission. When a case is discussed in an educational setting or a second opinion is sought, the clinician who first saw the patient in question should protect the privacy of the patient.

Application of Confidentiality

Conflicts and exceptions will arise surrounding the principle of confidentiality. There are instances when a provider can legally breach confidentiality. In certain situations, legal requirements exist to report diseases that can have an effect on the health of the public, such as sexually transmitted diseases. Reporting suspected child maltreatment (abuse and neglect), which is required as dental hygienists are mandated reporters in most states, is a violation of confidentiality. In dealing with minor children, divulging confidential information to the parents may be necessary to protect the child from harm. This is especially difficult with adolescents, who may or may not be adults according to the legal system. The patient's right to confidentiality often must be balanced against the rights of other individuals. In any situation, the healthcare provider must communicate to the patient the professional and legal responsibilities that exist for disclosure and work toward helping the patient as much as possible.

Fidelity is the belief that it is right to keep promises, be faithful, and fulfill commitments. Some philosophers consider this value as stemming from autonomy and the basic idea of respect for persons. Others denote it as a framework of confidentiality. For the healthcare provider, it includes the duty to fulfill all portions of expressed or **implied promises** made to the patient, in addition to holding to contractual agreements, not abandoning the patient before the completion of treatment, and keeping confidentiality.

Applying Principles and Values

Basic principles guide the dental hygienist and all healthcare providers in determining what is right and wrong in the practice of health care. From these principles are derived the rules laid out in all codes of ethics and codes of professional conduct. How these principles and codes are applied to decision making is the challenge for each healthcare provider faced with a professional problem or dilemma. What does a person do when duties conflict or when more than one principle is involved in a situation?

Prima Facie Duties

Thiroux[16] describes **prima facie duties** as duties that must be done before any other considerations enter the picture. *Prima facie* means "at first glance." Thiroux established two rules to deal with the conflict of prima facie duties:
1. Always do the act that is in accord with the stronger prima facie duty.
2. Always do the act that has the greatest of prima facie rightness over prima facie wrongness.

For example, the dental hygienist who suspects child maltreatment should place the welfare of the child over the autonomy of the parent. The stronger duty in this instance is the good of the child—beneficence—not the right of the parent.

These rules, with their supporting principles and values, can provide the dental hygienist guidance in the decision-making process. However, although these are good guides to use, they do not automatically provide correct ethical decisions because they sometimes are in conflict with each other. A choice must be made regarding which rule or value has precedence.

Summary

This chapter provides an introduction to the fundamental principles of ethics (nonmaleficence, beneficence, autonomy, justice) and several related values and concepts (paternalism, veracity, informed consent, confidentiality) commonly used to assist in ethical decision making. These principles and concepts are intellectual tools that can guide the dental hygienist in making difficult decisions when confronting an ethical dilemma or problem.

REFERENCES

1. Beauchamp TL, Childress J. *Principles of Biomedical Ethics*. 8th ed. Oxford University Press; 2019.
2. American Dental Association. The ADA Principles of Ethics and Code of Professional Conduct. 2020. https://www.ada.org/about/principles/code-of-ethics.
3. Merriam Webster's Dictionary. https://www.merriam-webster.com.
4. Frankena WK. *Ethics*. 2nd ed. Prentice-Hall; 1963.
5. Campbell CS, Rodgers VC. The normative principles of dental ethics. In Weinstein BD, ed. *Dental Ethics*. Lea & Febiger; 1993.
6. Rule JT, Veatch RM. *Ethical Questions in Dentistry*. 2nd ed. Quintessence; 2004.
7. Varkey B. Principles of clinical ethics and their application to practice. *Med Princ Pract*. 2020;30:17–28.
8. Velasquez M, Andre C, Shanks T, Meyer SJ, Meyer MJ. *Justice and Fairness*. Markkula Center for Applied Ethics at Santa Clara University; 2018. https://www.scu.edu/ethics/ethics-resources/ethical-decision-making/justice-and-fairness.
9. Kopelman L. On distinguishing justifiable from unjustifiable paternalism. *Virtual Mentor*. 2004;6(2):92–94. https://journalofethics.ama-assn.org/article/distinguishing-justifiable-unjustifiable-paternalism/2004-02.
10. Kahn JP, Hasegawa Jr TK. The dentist-patient relationship. In Weinstein BD, ed. *Dental Ethics*. Lea & Febiger; 1993.
11. Watterson DG. Informed consent and informed refusal in dentistry. *RDH*. 2012. https://www.rdhmag.com/patient-care/prosthodontics/article/16405751/informed-consent-and-informed-refusal-in-dentistry.
12. American Dental Association. *Managing Patients: Informed Consent/Refusal*. ADA Center for Professional Success; 2021.
13. Barstow C, Shahan B, Roberts M. Evaluating medical decision-making capacity in practice. *Am Fam Physician*. 2018;98(1):40–46.
14. Colby SL, Ortman, JM. Projections of the Size and Composition of the U.S. Population: 2014 to 2060. Population Estimates and Projections. Current Population Reports. United States Census Bureau; 2015. https://www.census.gov/content/dam/Census/library/publications/2015/demo/p25-1143.pdf.
15. Moyer J, Matson D. Assessment of decision-making capacity in older adults: an emerging area of practice and research. *J Gerontol B Psychol Sci Soc Sci*. 2007;62:3–11.
16. Thiroux JP, Krasemann KW. *Ethics Theory and Practice*. 11th ed. Pearson; 2015.

5

Codes of Ethics

KRISTIN MINIHAN-ANDERSON

LEARNING OUTCOMES

- Discuss the role of a code of ethics for the healthcare professions.
- Explain the value to the lay public of a professional code of ethics.
- Describe how a code of ethics can assist in the professional duty of self-regulation.
- Compare the 1927 version and the current version of the *ADHA Code of Ethics for Dental Hygienists*.
- List and describe the nine sections identified under the *Standards of Professional Responsibilities of the Code of Ethics for Dental Hygienists*.
- Be familiar with the code of the American Dental Association.

A **code of ethics** is one of the essential characteristics of a true profession. It is a guideline for members of a professional group used for self-regulation of the group. A major purpose of a **professional code** of ethics is to bind together the members of a group by expressing their goals and aspirations, as well as to define expected standards of behavior. The code is the contract the profession makes with society outlining the standards it will adhere to and uphold.

Professional Codes in Health Care

Ethical codes address the areas of personal integrity, dedication, and principled behavior.[1] Most healthcare providers cherish and hold sacred the obligations that flow from the entrance into their chosen profession. Acceptance and support of the prescribed principles and standards of behavior help reinforce the significance of being a part of a special group of people who are committed to the same values and goals.

Professional groups and the public have sometimes questioned the value of codes of ethics. Do codes of ethics really make a difference in the way healthcare providers interact with and treat patients and colleagues? If a member of a profession has seen evidence of colleagues acting unethically and those colleagues have not been punished, that question is legitimate. It would be the same for a member of the public who has had a bad experience with a healthcare provider. Patients may assume that they were treated in a manner inconsistent with the standards of behavior in the profession (even though the professional may have behaved appropriately). Sometimes the act may be inappropriate behavior by professionals; conversely, the frustration of patients may lead them to believe unethical behavior occurred even when it has not.

How, then, does a person know whether codes of ethics are ever effective? Three things demonstrate how codes can be effective in shaping professional behavior. First, when professional schools of healthcare screen applicants for admission to education programs, integrity and character are important criteria for acceptance. Admissions committees aim to select candidates who are the best qualified academically as well as candidates of good character. Virtue ethics, derived from the tradition of Plato and Aristotle, was introduced in Chapter 3. Virtue is a character trait; the assumption is that if someone is virtuous, they will act virtuously. Thus, part of the selection process often focuses on identifying virtue in the character of applicants.

Second, until proven otherwise, each entering student must be assumed to have the character traits needed to be a true professional. Educational institutions actively seek to indoctrinate students into the goals of the profession and expected professional behaviors. Learning what is expected of that professional person reinforces character traits in the developing professional. This often is accomplished by introducing students to the institution's code of conduct, by familiarizing them with the profession's code of ethics and professional conduct, by faculty serving as positive role models, and by enforcing adherence to expected professional behaviors when professional codes have been violated.

Third, after entering professional practice, it becomes the **obligation** of those professionals to help regulate their profession. When violations occur, members of the profession who become aware of these violations have a duty to intervene in a substantive way. This is a serious step and must be carefully considered; the reputation of the profession and the well-being of the public ultimately rest on a willingness to engage in meaningful self-policing of the profession.

The degree to which codes are effective remains a difficult question to answer completely. However, because health professions invest so much effort in the development and propagation of codes of ethics and standards of professional behavior, an assumption that the professions find them to be extremely valuable is reasonable. When violations of the code occur, the profession is empowered to take action to resolve the problem. Although codes alone do not guarantee that everyone will behave with integrity, they do provide guidance and standards by which professionals can be judged. Codes also serve as a touchstone by which all members of a profession can judge the acceptable parameters of behavior. This is why being a professional person is a privilege and carries both benefits and responsibilities.

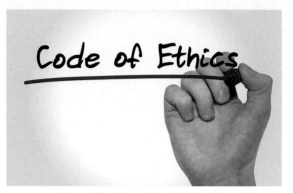

From: https://www.istockphoto.com.

Development of Ethical Codes

The first ethical code dates back to the time of the Greek physician Hippocrates, and the influence of the **Hippocratic Oath** is still reflected today in modern versions of ethical codes (Box 5.1). Traditional medical codes of ethics emphasize the physician's (1) duties in the individual patient–physician relationship, including the obligation of confidentiality, (2) authority and duty of beneficence (i.e., acting for the patient's good), and (3) obligation to each other.[2] In return for the power and prestige granted to the professions, a code of ethics is the promise to society to uphold certain values and standards in the practice of the profession. As noted, codes of ethics are aspirational in nature. They typically are powerful ethical statements, but they are not legal mandates. However, codes cannot easily be dismissed if there is a formal structure for self-regulation. In recent years, evidence has been increasing that state dental boards, which usually have authority over both dentists and dental hygienists, are sanctioning practitioners for legal violations as well as ethical violations. Because these boards typically have the authority to suspend or terminate a professional's right to practice, the fact that more attention is being given to ethical behavior makes the relationship between ethical codes and enforcement stronger. Ideally, codes should create a relationship among members of a profession that is similar to the ties in a family, obviating the need for enforcement outside the group. Additionally, there is often an inextricable link between the ethical and legal obligations of healthcare professionals. For example, a breach of confidentiality may constitute a breach

Hippocratic Oath

I swear by Apollo Physician and Asclepius and Hygeia and Panacea and all the gods and goddesses, making them my witnesses, that I will fulfill according to my ability and judgment this oath and this covenant:

To hold him who has taught me this art as equal to my parents and to live my life in partnership with him, and if he is in need of money to give him a share of mine, and to regard his offspring as equal to my brothers in male lineage and to teach them this art—if they desire to learn it—without fee and covenant; to give a share of precepts and oral instruction and all the other learning to my sons and to the sons of him who has instructed me and to pupils who have signed the covenant and have taken an oath according to the medical law, but no one else.

I will apply dietetic measures for the benefit of the sick according to my ability and judgment; I will keep them from harm and injustice.

I will neither give a deadly drug to anybody who asked for it, nor will I make a suggestion to this effect. Similarly I will not give to a woman an abortive remedy. In purity and holiness I will guard my life and my art.

I will not use the knife, not even on sufferers from stone, but will withdraw in favor of such men as are engaged in this work.

Whatever houses I may visit, I will come for the benefit of the sick, remaining free of all intentional injustice, of all mischief and in particular of sexual relations with both female and male persons, be they free or slaves.

What I may see or hear in the course of the treatment or even outside of the treatment in regard to the life of men, which on no account one must spread abroad, I will keep to myself, holding such things shameful to be spoken about.

If I fulfill this oath and do not violate it, may it be granted to me to enjoy life and art, being honored with fame among all men for all time to come; if I transgress it and swear falsely, may the opposite of all this be my lot.

special responsibility to the patients they treat because of their knowledge and the dependency of the patient on that knowledge. A code of ethics also is a set of commandments and, as such, has two principle functions. First, it provides an enforceable standard of minimally decent conduct for those who fall below that standard. Second, it indicates in general terms some of the ethical considerations a professional must consider when deciding on conduct.[4] The code of ethics can and does serve as a tool in the function of self-regulation.

The use of professional codes in health care has some limitations. Not every situation can be addressed in an ethical code or fully explained in an accompanying interpretation. Some philosophers have noted that most codes stress the obligations of healthcare professionals rather than describe the rights of those receiving healthcare services.[5] The current use of a patient's bill of rights in healthcare settings is an attempt to address this discrepancy.

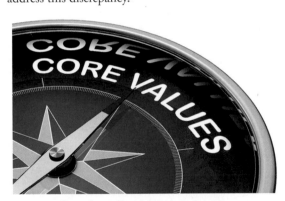

From: https://www.istockphoto.com.

Ethical Code for Dental Hygiene

The first code of ethics for dental hygienists was created at the inception of the American Dental Hygienists' Association (ADHA) in 1927.[6] The wording of the original code reflects the tone and verbiage of the time and the fact that initially, only women were dental hygienists. That code, developed in three sections that list the duties of the profession to patients, reads as follows:

Section 1: *The dental hygienist should be ever ready to respond to the wants of her patrons, and should fully recognize the obligations involved in the discharge of*

of the Health Insurance Portability and Accountability Act (HIPAA), which could incur legal liability. Professionals' obligations to each other, to patients, and to society should be similar to the strong obligations and emotional feelings that attend belonging to a family, with the behavior of members being monitored by the membership.

A sound and deep understanding of the moral responsibilities of those entrusted with the health of others is essential.[3] Healthcare providers have a *her duties toward them. As she is in most cases unable to correctly estimate the character of her operations, her own sense of right must guarantee faithfulness in their performance. Her manner should be firm, yet kind and sympathizing so as to gain the respect and confidence of her patients, and even the simplest case committed to her care should receive that attention which is due to operations performed on living, sensitive tissue.*

*   **Section 2:** It is not to be expected that the patient will possess a very extended or very accurate knowledge of professional matters. The dental hygienist should make due allowance for this, patiently explaining many things which seem quite clear to herself, thus endeavoring to educate the public mind so that it will properly appreciate the beneficent efforts of our profession. She should encourage no false hopes by promising success when in the nature of the case there is uncertainty.*

*   **Section 3:** The dental hygienist should be temperate in all things, keeping both mind and body in the best possible health, that her patients may have the benefit of the clearness of judgment and skill which is their right.*

The code has been revised several times over the years, most significantly in 1995 after a thoughtful review and the incorporation of newer aspects of health care and changes in the profession. Minor revisions have been undertaken in more recent years. This version of the code is presented in several sections and encompasses the areas of endeavor in which the dental hygienist functions. The purpose, illustrated by four objectives of the code of ethics, is listed in the beginning of the code, and these capture the essence of why the code is important to dental hygienists and the public who entrust themselves for care and services. The key concepts, basic beliefs, fundamental principles, and core values are established and explained in the code so that the standards of professional responsibility can be fully understood by professionals and public alike.

For dental hygienist students, the code of ethics for dental hygienists is a vehicle for educating novices about the obligations of the profession, informing them about the basic beliefs and fundamental principles of the group, and providing guidelines regarding the expected behavior of a dental hygiene practitioner. The topic of ethics is usually integrated throughout the dental hygienist entry-level curriculum both didactically and clinically. The American Dental Association's Commission on Dental Accreditation (CODA), the agency that sets the standards for all dental health-related education programs, requires graduates of accredited dental hygienist programs to be "competent in the application of the principles of ethical reasoning, ethical decision making and professional responsibility as they pertain to the academic environment, research, patient care, and practice management."[7]

All professional codes are evolving documents that embody the contract between a particular profession and the public. For dental hygienists, the code is maintained by the professional organization (the ADHA) and is monitored by the executive staff of the organization. When deemed necessary, the officers of the association appoint a committee of members to review and revise the document. The code can be amended at any meeting of the ADHA House of Delegates by a two-thirds vote of that group. The ADHA and all healthcare professional organizations have, as a condition of membership, an agreement to uphold the profession's code of ethics.

The code of ethics that was first developed in 1995 is more comprehensive than earlier versions and provides extensive guidance for the dental hygienist working in a variety of healthcare delivery settings. The current code lists the core principles embraced and upheld in all healthcare professions and clearly defines all the standards of professional responsibility that the ADHA believes its members should adhere to in the performance of their services. A code of ethics is a reference and a guide. It should be studied by students and referred to for guidance by working professionals (Figure 5.1). The ADHA *Code of Ethics for Dental Hygienists* can be found on the organization's website (https://www.adha.org), the Core Values are presented in Table 5.1.[8]

The dental hygienist is most often an employee of a dentist. Individuals employed by a dentist should be familiar with not only the ADHA Code of Ethics but also the ADA code.

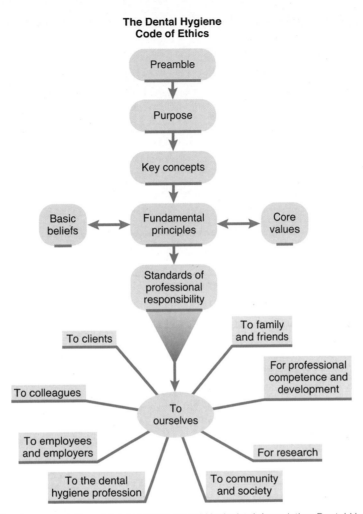

The Dental Hygiene Code of Ethics

- **Fig. 5.1** Visual representation of the American Dental Hygienists' Association *Dental Hygiene Code of Ethics*. Although the specific language of the code has been updated through the years, its basic components and aims remain the same. From: American Dental Hygienists' Association. *The Dental Hygiene Code of Ethics*, as appeared in the January 1995 issue of *Access* magazine. Reproduced with permission of American Dental Hygienists' Association in the format Textbook via Copyright Clearance Center.

Summary

Codes of ethics are the written standards to which healthcare professionals agree to adhere before society, which grants certain privileges to these groups. Among these privileges are societal trust and self-regulation. Once individuals have gained the necessary professional knowledge and skill and acquired their professional license, which is an acknowledgment of this achievement, they are accorded professional status. The responsibility that goes with this status is to uphold the core values of the profession of dental hygienists: professional autonomy, confidentiality, societal trust, nonmaleficence, beneficence, justice, and veracity.

resolution of ethical dilemmas. Odom was the first to report that the usual approach to teaching ethics in dental and dental hygiene schools is either the lecture format or the lecture and case analysis format.[1] He, as well as others, have suggested and supported the concept that students need opportunities to develop the analytical skills needed to assess ethical dilemmas. Odom further suggested that posing ethical dilemma cases when a panel of experts is available to help students analyze and arrive at possible solutions to the hypothetical dilemmas is a means of affording those opportunities.[2,3] Kacerik et al. found that ethics was overwhelmingly (98%) taught in the didactic component of the curriculum in dental hygiene programs with far fewer hours devoted to the clinical application of theory.[4] This oftentimes leaves dental hygienists feeling ill-equipped to handle ethical dilemmas they may encounter in the workplace.

The teaching of ethics in dental and dental hygiene educational programs has been acknowledged as an essential part of the education of the dental healthcare professional. As mentioned in Chapter 5, the CODA Accreditation Standards for Dental Hygiene Education Programs dictates that "Graduates must be competent in the application of the principles of ethical reasoning, ethical decision making, and professional responsibility as they pertain to the academic environment, research, patient care, and practice management."[5] However, these accreditation standards simply provide general guidelines—dental hygiene programs vary related to hours spent didactically and clinically on this topic.

In 1989, the American Dental Education Association (ADEA) established guidelines for all dental-related educational programs that stated that curricula should provide opportunities for refining skills of **ethical analysis** so students are able to apply ethical principles to new and emerging problems in the profession. The goal for these curricula was to develop a commitment by the students to the **moral principles** that are the basis of the profession's contract with society. The ADEA policy has been revised since that time to include expanded statements on professional behavior, societal obligations, access to care needs, and community service.[6] Within the Core Competencies domain of the Competencies for Entry into the Profession of Dental Hygiene published by the ADEA, "apply a professional Code of Ethics in all endeavors" is listed first.[7]

Intellectual and clinical skills are essential to the competent provision of oral health care, which is why ethics and professionalism are required in the dental hygiene educational curricula. Effectively fostering and evaluating the ability of students in ethical reasoning and critical thinking are challenging tasks. When faculty are trained in ethical reasoning skills and the authentic evaluation of students, the outcomes are positive, faculty are more comfortable evaluating professional judgment, and students report being competent in the skills.[8,9]

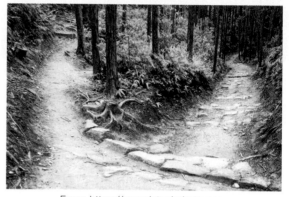

From: https://www.istockphoto.com.

Ethical Awareness

How the dental hygienist responds to ethical issues that arise in practice depends on the ethical awareness of the individual (**moral sensitivity**). A situation or problem can be perceived by one individual as having an ethical component but not by another. Campbell and Rogers categorized the kind of moral problems encountered in life and dental practice (Table 6.1).[10] Their first category deals with problems of **moral weakness**, in which moral responsibilities point in one direction and personal inclinations in another. The dental hygienist who forgoes providing a patient with needed dental health education because he or she wants to get to lunch early is lacking in professional responsibility. Another category is **moral uncertainty**, which is defined as the question of whether a moral obligation exists and its scope. For a dental hygienist, dealing with a noncompliant periodontal patient could raise issues of uncertainty. How far should the dental hygienist go to attain a level of health when the patient is unwilling or uninterested in following good dental

TABLE 6.1	Categories of Moral Problems
Category	Characteristic
Moral weakness	Moral responsibilities conflict with personal inclinations.
Moral uncertainty	The question is whether a moral obligation exists.
Moral dilemma	Obligations and responsibilities are in conflict.
Moral distress	Frustration results from perceived powerlessness when what is happening appears to be wrong and one cannot to act ethically.

Data from: Campbell CS, Rogers VC. The normative principles of dental ethics. In: Weinstein BD, ed. *Dental Ethics.* Lea & Febiger; 1993.

TABLE 6.2	The "Four A's" to Rise Above Moral Distress
Term	Description
Ask	Ask about distress. Are you showing signs of work-related distress? Become aware of the problem.
Affirm	Affirm your distress and the commitment to take care of yourself. Affirm the professional obligation to act.
Assess	Identify sources of distress and determine severity. Analyze risks and benefits.
Act	Prepare personally and professionally to take action.

Data from: American Association of Critical Care Nurses. *AACN Public Policy Position Statement: Moral Distress.* AACN; 2008.

health advice and guidance? The third category is composed of problems that are **moral dilemmas.** A moral dilemma exists when obligations or responsibilities are in conflict. A large portion of the bioethics literature deals with moral dilemmas that often involve matters of life and death.

Moral Distress

The term **moral distress** is included here to acknowledge situations in which the healthcare provider is frustrated by feelings of powerlessness when a perceived wrong is occurring but is unable to act. It is the feeling experienced when—because of a system issue, the resistance of a powerful person, or a restraint in the situation—an individual cannot do what is believed to be what ought to be done. The use of this term came from the nursing profession and describes situations in which the nurse feels powerless to act ethically.[11,12] Although this is a newer term, the resulting distress, emotional toll, anger, guilt, and depression are familiar to many healthcare providers who must balance conflicts of conscience with professional expectations. An example of this for the dental hygienist could be when treatment recommended by another provider for a patient is deemed excessive or unnecessary. The American Association of Critical Care Nurses (AACCN) advocates a model for rising above moral distress called the "four A's."[13] The goal of this model is to preserve the integrity and authenticity of the healthcare provider. Addressing moral distress requires making changes (Table 6.2).

Morally courageous professionals are encouraged to persevere in standing up for what is right even when it means they may do so alone. Murray provided a listing of seven critical checkpoints to use in ethical decision making.[14] His guiding checkpoints start with evaluating the need for moral courage and end with avoiding what might restrain moral courage. In a clinical setting, whether it is a small or large group of practitioners, there can be an unwillingness to face the challenge of addressing unethical behaviors. Those who have the courage to stand up and speak out need the support of their peers.

The following are checkpoints to apply in ethical decision making:
- Evaluate the circumstances to establish whether moral courage is needed in the situation.
- Determine what moral values and ethical principles are at risk or in the question of being compromised.
- Ascertain what principles must be expressed and defended in the situation. Focus on one or two of the more critical values.
- Consider the possible adverse consequences and risks associated with taking action.

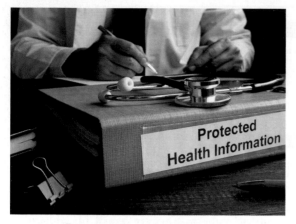

From: https://www.istockphoto.com.

5. Make the Decision

When each alternative has been clearly outlined in terms of pros and cons, a reasonable framework is apparent for making a decision. Each option must then be considered in turn, with attention to how many pros and cons would attend each decision. The seriousness of the cons must then be weighed by the dental hygienist, remembering that, as a professional, he or she is obliged to put the patient's interests first. Simply by examining the options in a careful way, the best solution to an ethical dilemma frequently becomes obvious. Before implementing the decision, the practitioner should replay each principle against the decision to see if the decision holds up to this evaluation.

6. Implement the Decision

The final step involves acting on the decision that has been made. The decision process will have been futile if no action is taken. Many appropriate decisions are never implemented because this step is omitted. Remember that no action represents tacit approval of a situation.

Ethical Dilemmas for the Dental Hygienist

The dental hygienist may be faced with a wide variety of ethical issues and moral dilemmas. A few studies have addressed the responsibility of dental hygienists to report unethical practices. In 1990 Gaston and colleagues conducted a survey of ethical issues in dental hygiene.[16] They found that the three most frequently encountered practice dilemmas were observation of

behavior in conflict with standard infection control procedures, failure to refer patients to a specialist, and nondiagnosis of dental disease. One of the conclusions drawn from this study was that serious ethical dilemmas are encountered by most dental hygienists, prompting the authors to advocate for increased education of hygienists in the recognition and resolution of ethical problems.

The range and type of ethical problems have continued to expand, and because most hygienists are employees, issues around employment are commonplace. Unfair treatment involving assignments of hours, compensation, benefits, unsafe work environment, and noncompliance with state or federal regulations are reported by dental hygienists.[17]

Dentistry, unlike medicine, usually is performed in small or large group practices in which little, if any, institutional oversight is provided by groups such as ethics committees or standard review boards. Dental hygienists usually are employed by a dentist or a group of dentists. This arrangement can place the hygienist in a difficult situation when inappropriate care or unethical practices are observed, especially when the dentist's employer is involved in the action. In these situations, if the dental hygienist advocates for the good of the patient, continued employment may be in jeopardy—thus causing moral distress. Conversely, if the hygienist remains silent, professionalism is compromised and no one speaks for the interests of the patient. This dilemma is similar to what many registered nurses are subjected to when they become advocates for a hospitalized patient.[18] A conflict or dilemma can be intensified when a subordinate observes an unethical action performed by an individual in a position of power. Studies from the nursing literature have reported such situations having a negative influence on the healthcare environment and leading to burnout and departure from the profession.[18,19] Any type of an ethical dilemma or problem can arise in the practice of dental hygiene. Box 6.1 lists the categories of ethical dilemmas most frequently encountered by dental hygienists.

Additional types of dilemmas and problems can and will arise. Major advances in technology and the changes in delivery and payment systems in dentistry will further alter the scope and depth of ethical challenges facing dental hygienists and dentists.

<table>
<tr><td>• BOX 6.1</td><td>Categories of Ethical Dilemmas Most Commonly Encountered by Dental Hygienists</td></tr>
</table>

1. Substandard Care
   Situations in which there is failure to diagnose, failure to refer, or lack of proper infection control or in which dental or dental hygiene services are provided that do not meet the accepted standard of care.
2. Overtreatment
   Situations in which excessive services or services that are unnecessary for a particular case are provided. This category includes unduly influencing a patient's care decision as a result of one's position of greater knowledge.
3. Scope of Practice
   Instances in which the legally assigned scope of practice is exceeded by a dental hygienist, dentist, or other member of the dental team.
4. Fraud
   Situations in which an insurance claim or other reimbursement mechanism is adjusted to favor the dental office or the patient's financial situation. Other types of false charting or other cost-containment efforts may be included in this category.
5. Confidentiality Breaches
   Situations in which patient and/or child–parent confidentiality is jeopardized or the need and requirement for informed consent is not met.
6. Impaired Professional
   Situations in which the dental hygienist or other dental team member cannot or should not perform appropriate dental care because of a dependence on alcohol, drugs, or other substances (**impaired professional**).
7. Sexual Harassment
   Includes a wide range of behaviors that a dental team member may observe or be subjected to that can be classified as harassment.
8. Abuse
   Situations in which abuse of a child, elder, or spouse is observed or suspected. Such situations have legal requirements as well as ethical considerations in most states.

Dental hygienists also are increasingly finding employment in areas other than private practice, such as research, public health, and corporate fields. These arenas will pose different ethical dilemmas for these individuals.

Solving a Dilemma Using the Ethical Decision-Making Model

The following hypothetical case is an example of a typical ethical dilemma often faced by a dental hygienist in a private practice situation. This case is presented to illustrate how the ethical decision-making model can be applied to an ethical dilemma.

Joan Lakeside is a dental hygienist who graduated last year from a dental hygiene program near her hometown. Since graduation, she has been working for a dentist, Dr. Tom McVey, who has been practicing for 20 years. The practice is growing, and Dr. McVey is happy to have Joan working 4 days a week in his busy office. He often tells her how pleased he is with her work and comments how lucky they both were to attend State University Dental School, one of the best in the country.

A patient of the practice, Steve Stafford, is scheduled for an appointment with Joan for the first time. Steve is a 51-year-old White male with normal vital signs, no current medications, and no history of systemic disease. His periodontal condition is good overall, but he does occasionally smoke cigars. Joan notices a small, indurated, white and reddish, slightly raised lesion on the right side of Steve's tongue. On questioning her patient, Joan finds out that he is unaware of the lesion or how long it has been present in his mouth. Joan shows the lesion to Dr. McVey when he comes into the room to chat with Steve. In earshot of the patient, Dr. McVey tells Joan, "Not to worry. It is nothing. We'll take a look at it in six or seven months, or whenever Steve gets back in here for his next cleaning."

At the end of the day, Joan goes into Dr. McVey's office and shares with him her concern that the lesion in Steve's mouth looks suspicious and should be referred for biopsy. Once again, Dr. McVey tells her not to worry, adding "It is my decision as to whether or not we send Steve for a biopsy." Joan is very uncomfortable about the situation and wonders if she should call the patient directly to advise him to seek further examination regarding the lesion on his tongue.

Step 1 in the ethical decision-making model is to identify the dilemma. Joan is concerned about her patient and believes that the lesion on his tongue may be cancerous. Her employer tells her not to be concerned because he does not believe the lesion requires immediate attention. Joan is not reassured because she recalls seeing slides in her pathology class that resemble the lesion on Steve's tongue. Should she call the patient and tell him to seek further examination, or simply forget it and wait until he comes in for his next appointment? That is Joan's ethical dilemma—to call the patient or not.

Steps 2 and 3 involve gathering all pertinent information and listing possible options for action. Joan checks in her oral pathology book and confirms that the lesion on Steve's tongue looks very much like the photographs of squamous cell carcinoma in her text. She identifies the following as her options:

1. Go back to Dr. McVey with her textbook, and restate her suspicions in an attempt to convince him to refer the patient for a diagnostic biopsy.
2. Call the patient directly and advise him to seek another opinion about his lesion.
3. Do nothing and wait until the patient comes in for his next appointment.

Step 4 requires that Joan apply the ethical principles and rules to each option she has identified. Option 1—talking to Dr. McVey and convincing him to call the patient in for another examination—applies the principles of nonmaleficence and autonomy. Removing harm is in the patient's best interest, which, in this case, is a possibly cancerous lesion. Option 2—calling the patient directly and advising him to seek care for the lesion—applies the principles of autonomy and beneficence. Autonomy is involved because the patient came in for an examination and has a right to know that he may or may not have a disease. Beneficence—doing good for the patient—is applicable because doing nothing could cause the patient great harm if the lesion were found to be cancerous. Option 3—doing nothing and waiting for 6 or 7 months—may involve respecting the autonomy of the dentist.

After completing steps 1 through 4, Joan is prepared for step 5: the decision stage. Joan decides to approach Dr. McVey again and try to convince him to call the patient in for another appointment. If she is unsuccessful in convincing her employer, she will call the patient directly.

Step 6 is implementation. Joan resolves to speak to Dr. McVey first thing the next morning.

The process of ethical decision making can be facilitated by using the decision-making model just described. Numerous other models can be applied to problem solving. Many healthcare workers find that talking to trusted colleagues and peers about ethical dilemmas and work problems can be both beneficial and comforting. The ethical decision-making model can be applied in a small group and is equally effective for students and experienced practitioners. A sample of a worksheet for assisting in the decision-making process is provided in Figure 6.2.

Summary

Ethical choices and dilemmas inevitably occur during the career of any healthcare professional. Ethical decision making, like other aspects of dental hygiene care, is learned during the education of the dental hygienist and then applied in the practice of dental hygiene. The use of an ethical decision-making model can help the healthcare professional think through an ethical dilemma and arrive at a decision. The six-step model presented in this chapter can provide structure and guide the dental hygienist when faced with an ethical dilemma.

PRACTICE POINTER

Use the six-step model when faced with an ethical dilemma in the workplace. This will assist the dental hygienist to arrive at an ethically sound decision and aid in avoiding potential liability.

REFERENCES

1. Odom JG. The status of dental ethics instruction. *J Dent Educ.* 1988;52:306.

2. Odom JG. Recognizing and resolving ethical dilemmas in dentistry. *Med Law.* 1985;4:543.

3. Odom JG, Beemsterboer PL, Pate T, Haden NK. Revisiting the status of dental ethics instruction. *J Dent Educ.* 2000;64:772.

4. Kacerik MG, Prajer RG, Conrad C. Ethics instruction in the dental hygiene curriculum. *J Dental Hygiene.* 2006;80(1):9.

5. Commission on Dental Accreditation (CODA). Accreditation Standards for Dental Hygiene Education Programs. 2022. https://legacy.ada.org/en/coda/current-accreditation-standards. Accessed September 29, 2021.

6. American Dental Education Association. ADEA policy statements. *J Dent Educ.* 2014;78:1057.

7. American Dental Education Association. Competencies for entry into the allied dental professions. 2011. https://www.adea.org/about_adea/governance/documents/competency-docs2011.pdf. Accessed September 29, 2021.

8. Christie CR, Bowen DM, Paarmann CS. Curriculum evaluation of ethical reasoning and professional responsibility. *J Dent Educ.* 2003;67:55.

9. Christie CR, Bowen DM, Paarmann CS. Effectiveness of faculty training to enhance clinical evaluation of student competence in ethical reasoning and professionalism. *J Dent Educ.* 2007;71:1048.

10. Campbell CS, Rogers VC. The normative principles of dental ethics editor. In: Weinstein BD, ed. *Dental Ethics.* Lea & Febiger; 1993.

11. Corley MC. Nurse moral distress: a proposed theory and research agenda, *Nurs Ethics.* 2002;9:636.

12. Hamric AB, David WS, Childress MD. Moral distress in health care professionals: what is it and what can we do about it? *Pharos Alpha Omega Alpha Honor Med Soc.* 2006;69(1):16–23.

13. American Association of Critical-Care Nurses. AACN Public Policy Position Statement: Moral Distress. AACN; 2008.

14. Murray JS. Moral courage in healthcare: acting ethically even in the presence of risk. *Online J Issues Nurs.* 2010;15:3. https://ojin.nursingworld.org/MainMenuCategories/EthicsStandards/Resources/Courage-and-Distress/Moral-Courage-and-Risk.html.

15. Jonsen AR, Siegler M, Winslade WJ. *Clinical Ethics: A Practical Approach to Ethical Decisions in Clinical Medicine.* 7th ed. McGraw-Hill, 2010.

16. Gaston MA, Brown DM, Waring MB. Survey of ethical issues in dental hygiene. *J Dent Hyg.* 1990;64:216.

17. Majeski J. Ethical issues for the dental hygienist. *Access.* 2013;27:16–20.

18. Redman B, Fry ST. Nurses' ethical conflicts: what is really known about them? *Nurs Ethics.* 2000;7:360.

19. Kalvemark S, Hoglund AT, Hansson MG, Westerholm P, Arnetz B. Living with conflicts: ethical dilemmas and moral distress in the health care system. *Soc Sci Med.* 2004;58A:1075.

7

Social Responsibility

FRANK CATALANOTTO AND KRISTIN MINIHAN-ANDERSON

CHAPTER OUTLINE

LEARNING OUTCOMES

- Describe the role of the dental hygienist in meeting the oral healthcare needs of the public.
- Relate the importance of the *Surgeon General's Report on Oral Health* to the profession of dental hygiene.
- List several facts about oral health disparities in America.
- Describe the issue of access to care and social responsibility.
- Describe dental therapists and their role in addressing access to dental care.
- Identify several strategies that a dental hygienist can implement in striving for social justice.

The dental hygienist assumes the rights and responsibilities of service in the greater good as a healthcare provider and a professional. This chapter reviews the issues of disparity in oral healthcare, access to care, and the responsibilities of all oral healthcare professionals to advocate the just distribution of resources to meet the oral healthcare needs of the public.

In his March 1966 presentation to the Committee on Human Rights Dr. Martin Luther King made the following statement: "Of all forms of inequality, injustice in health care is the most shocking and inhumane."

Disparities in Oral Health Care

Surgeon General's Report on Oral Health

The first *Surgeon General's Report on Oral Health* was published in the year 2000. Major findings are listed in Box 7.1. This landmark report described the meaning of oral health and explained why oral health is essential to general health and well-being.[1] The use of the term *oral health* and not *dental health* was a deliberate choice because oral health means more than healthy teeth. The report included conditions and diseases such as oral cancers, lesions of the head and neck, birth defects, and facial pain. The phrase "the mouth is a mirror" of the body was used to emphasize the oral-systemic connection as it relates to disease. The report established the reciprocal relationship between oral health and general health and that the two should not be looked at separately. Oral health is a critical component of overall health.

The surgeon general's report also addressed the disparities and inequalities that affect the most vulnerable populations: the poor, children, the elderly, the disabled, and racial and ethnic minorities. These groups often cannot access care for financial reasons, but lack

- Oral diseases and disorders affect health and well-being throughout life.
- Safe and effective measures exist to prevent common oral diseases.
- The mouth reflects general health and well-being.
- Oral diseases and conditions are associated with other health problems.
- Lifestyle behaviors that affect general health affect oral and craniofacial health.
- Profound and consequential oral health disparities are present in the population of the United States.
- More information is needed to improve oral health and eliminate health disparities.
- Research is the key to a further reduction in the burden of diseases and disorders that affect the craniofacial complex.

Data from: U.S. Department of Health and Human Services. *Oral Health in America: A Report of the Surgeon General*. National Institutes of Health; 2000.

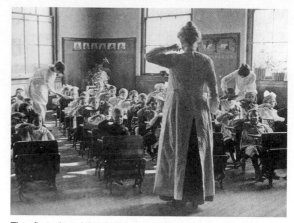

The first dental hygienists provided oral health education in public schools in Bridgeport, CT. Courtesy: University of Bridgeport, Fones School of Dental Hygiene.

exist among lower-income adults and those in particular geographic areas, and the cost is a major obstacle to Americans obtaining necessary dental care.[2]

Oral Health Disparities

The National Institute of Dental and Craniofacial Research addressed the disparity issue by publishing *A Plan to Eliminate Craniofacial, Oral and Dental Health Disparities* in 2002.[3] This report listed many factors besides finances that must be identified when determining why certain populations become patients and others do not. By 2050, racial and ethnic minority groups are expected to no longer be "minorities" but will constitute the emerging majority of the population of the United States. Social, political, economic, and cultural factors clearly underlie the complex social problem of inequality. Although these problems are not new, they continue to confound and frustrate.

The Centers for Disease Control and Prevention (CDC) provides data and resources outlining how sociodemographic factors are significant risk indicators for poor oral health:[4]

- Sex: Men experience head and neck cancers at twice the rate of women.
- Race/ethnicity: Untreated dental caries significantly impact members of particular racial and ethnic groups of all ages.
- Socioeconomic status (SES): Previous research has identified a strong association between low SES

of access also can be caused by fear and complex psychosocial or cultural assumptions. How to address this need is a social responsibility of all healthcare professionals working with public and private agencies. It is a complex and challenging problem in which the dental hygienist is well suited to be an active participant.

The publication of the 2020 Surgeon General's Report *Oral Health in America: Advances and Challenges* sought to provide answers regarding the current state of oral health, advances made since the 2000 report, challenges that persist since the last report, threats that are new and/or emerging, and promising new directions for research and oral health improvement. The guiding principle of the 2020 report is "The report will describe and evaluate oral health and the interaction between oral health and general health throughout the lifespan, considering advances in science, healthcare integration, and social influences to articulate promising new directions for improving oral health and oral health equity across communities."

Introductory documents of this publication indicate the following: many of the oral health disparities and access problems discussed in 2000 are still present today, the aging population in the United States is experiencing less edentulism although disparities still and the severity and prevalence of oral diseases. Oral diseases disproportionally impact children and adults from low-income households.

- Age: Periodontitis in older adults (65+ years) occurs at a rate of 60% compared to a rate of 42% in younger adults.

The deaths of two children from dental abscesses made headlines in 2006 and triggered some legislative actions to attempt to prevent similar tragedies.[5] Recent reports document that the death of Deamonte Driver, one of the children referenced here, was not an isolated event and that there are significant morbidities and mortality associated with severe dental problems such as dental infections.[6,7]

Health Disparities and Professionalism

As a society, we are faced with disparities in health care and in dental health care. More than 30 million people in the United States under the age of 65 are estimated to have no health insurance; this is a great concern for the public health and well-being of the country.[8] It has been estimated that over 190,000,000 Americans do not access dental care on a regular basis.[9,10] Approximately 60,000,000 Americans live in **Dental Health Professional Shortage Areas (DHPSA)**.[11]

Dental hygienists are focused on prevention, a focus that fits well with the goals of health promotion that have been established by the US Department of Health and Human Services and with the lack of access to dental care and the resulting oral health disparities previously noted. Two subsequent reports called for significant expansion of the role of dental hygienists in meeting the challenges of oral health-care disparities. In celebrating the 100th anniversary of the dental hygiene profession, in 2013 the ADHA published a report entitled "Transforming Dental Hygiene Education and the Profession for the 21st Century"[12]; this report called for significant change in both the education and future role of the dental hygienist in the oral healthcare workforce. At about the same time, the National Governors Association issued a brief entitled "The Role of Dental Hygienists in Providing Access to Oral Health Care"[13]; again, this report called attention to the role of dental hygienists in addressing access to care, particularly for underserved patients. These reports lay the foundation for both oral healthcare workforce policy changes but also a reminder of the ethical commitments of dental hygienists as oral healthcare professionals.

The responsibility of all oral healthcare professionals to assist and lead society in finding solutions to oral **health disparities** is based on the historic definition of a profession.[14] This concept of service and the aspirations for professionalism in dental hygiene are established in the code of ethics and addressed in its fundamental principles and core values. Listed under the ADHA Code of Ethics as well as the *Standards of Professional Responsibility, to the Community and Society*[15] are several points that include increasing access to care, promoting public health, supporting justice, and recognizing an obligation to provide pro bono service. As a group, dental hygienists aspire to make a contribution to the public and to enhance all the ability to seek and receive dental care resources. Dental care is, by its nature, a social enterprise even when normally provided on a one-on-one basis.[16] The **social contract** made between the public and healthcare professionals, such as dental hygienists and dentists, is the basis of this relationship.

Dental hygienists and dentists take pride in being recognized as professional healthcare providers. Welie, in a series of articles examining what it means to be a professional, defined a profession as a "collective of expert services providers who have jointly and publicly committed to always give priority to the existential needs and interests of the public they serve ahead of their own and who in turn are trusted by the public to do so".[17–19] Thus, the benefit of being called a professional also carries the burden of addressing the needs of the public. How the dental hygienist uses his or her skills and knowledge to advance the public good is part of the obligation laid out in the code of ethics and embraced in the essence of a professional person. We must consider our obligations as a group, not just individuals who are members of a group, by honoring the justice principle in the code of ethics and sharing ethical concerns as a moral community.[20,21]

Ethical Goals in Oral Health Care

The values of caring, stewardship, and justice are of great importance for achieving ethical goals in healthcare—they are the goals that focus on society. These are

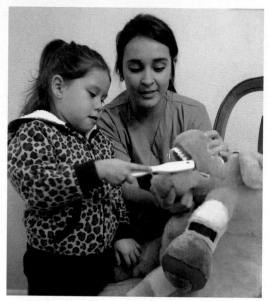

Courtesy: Nichole Salazar.

different from the ethical principles that focus on the individual, such as autonomy and self-determination.

Justice in dental care is a complex topic. What is just or fair? What does the just distribution of dental healthcare resources look like? For the parents of a child with a toothache who can find a dentist and pay for dental services, no dilemma exists. For the parents of a child with a toothache who cannot find a dentist because they have no ability to pay for services or have no access to a public program, a dilemma certainly exists, as does the need to examine the disparities of the situation. As discussed in Chapter 4, *distributive justice* is the term used when discussing allocation of resources in large social systems. Saying that everyone should have access to dental care is easy, but what kind of care are individuals entitled to when resources are limited? The first response might be basic dental care or adequate dental care. Defining what that might be is a daunting task that challenges communities and the federal government. Even the term *access* can be misleading, with access defined as the freedom or ability to obtain health care, and *accessibility* defined as the ease with which health care can be reached in the face of barriers such as finance or culture.[22] As Garetto and Yoder stated, we also have a responsibility to those who are unaware of need, do not seek it, cannot get to it, or are afraid of it.[23] Ethically, the goal of improving

the health of the population is a societal greater good benefiting society at large.

Social Justice

Numerous authors and national reports have addressed the importance of teaching social responsibility as part of professionalism. Two reports from the Institute of Medicine (IOM) in the early 2000s advocated increased professionalism and **social justice** as a part of improving quality and bridging the gaps in health care.[24,25] The American Dental Education Association (ADEA) defined its role and responsibility with its member institutions in improving the oral health status of all Americans in a report in 2003 and is now an established association policy (Box 7.2).[26] The findings stressed the importance of increasing the diversity of the oral healthcare workforce and teaching and exhibiting values that prepare future dental professionals to commit to delivering oral healthcare to all populations, including the underserved. The message from the healthcare professions is that professionalism includes social responsibility, an ethic of caring, and access to that care for all members of society.[27]

> **• BOX 7.2** **American Dental Education Association Recommendations for Improving the Oral Health Status of All Americans**
>
> Roles and Responsibilities of Academic Dental Institutions:
>
> - Monitor future oral healthcare workforce needs.
> - Improve the effectiveness of the oral healthcare delivery system.
> - Prepare students to provide oral healthcare services to diverse populations.
> - Increase the diversity of the oral healthcare workforce.
> - Improve the effectiveness of allied dental professionals in reaching the underserved.
>
> Modified from: Haden NK, Catalanotto FA, Alexander CJ, Bailit H, Battrell A, Broussard J Jr, Buchanan J, Douglass CW, Fox CE 3rd, Glassman P, Lugo RI, George M, Meyerowitz C, Scott ER 2nd, Yaple N, Bresch J, Gutman-Betts Zlata, Luke GG, Moss M, Sinkford JC, Weaver RG, Valachovic RW, ADEA. Improving the oral health status of all Americans: Roles and Responsibilities of Academic Dental Institutions: The Report of the ADEA President's Commission. *J Dent Educ.* 2003;67:563.

Dental Therapists as Part of the Oral Healthcare Workforce

Dental therapists are a relatively recent addition to the oral healthcare team in the United States. Dental therapists have been utilized for over 100 years in over 50 countries. They were first introduced in the United States in Alaska in 2002 to provide dental care to indigenous populations. Their introduction was met with fierce resistance by the American Dental Association and affiliated state organizations, but dental therapy legislation has been passed by 12 states with several other states considering such legislation.[28] Although there have been unsupported claims about safety, quality of care, and cost-effectiveness of dental therapists in providing dental care, especially to underserved populations, all the published evidence strongly counters these concerns.[29,30] In addition, in 2015 the American Dental Association's Commission on Dental Accreditation (CODA) approved accreditation standards for dental therapy educational programs[31] that include 3 years of education. However, dental hygienists can receive credit for their existing education as "advanced standing" and can usually accomplish the necessary additional education to become a dental therapist in about 18 months of additional training.[32]

Challenges to Ethical Practice and Social Justice and the Role of the Dental Hygienist

A dentist's decision to participate or not in safety net programs such as Medicaid can be viewed as a fulfillment of the *social contract* and maintaining a *social justice* perspective. For example, a paper by McKernan and colleagues showed that Iowa dentists who participated in that state's Medicaid program scored significantly higher in altruistic attitudes.[33] Similarly, a paper by Logan and colleagues showed that dentists who participated in Florida's Medicaid program felt a sense of social stigma from other dentists who did not participate in Medicaid.[34] Because only 26.4% of dentists nationally accept Medicaid patients,[35] this can pose a challenge for the dental hygienist who believes in a social justice perspective.

Most dental hygienists work in an employer/employee setting in which a solo dentist or small group of dentists owns and manages the dental care business.

What can a dental hygienist do to fulfill a commitment to social justice? It is not prudent or feasible for a dental hygienist employee in such a situation to provide free or discounted dental hygiene care; this kind of "Band-Aid" approach would not solve the greater problem anyway.[36,37] However, the dental hygienist can be a part of the movement to alleviate disparities and develop effective care systems in many other ways.

The following are some suggested activities to address these societal disparities:

- Provide dental hygiene services at a safety net clinic.
- Work on a community campaign to install fluoridation in the local water district.
- Participate in state-organized caries prevention programs.
- Work with local dental groups to address oral health disparities.
- Support school-based fluoride and sealant programs.
- Volunteer at general and dental health fairs.
- Provide dental hygiene services in mobile dental vans.
- Support collaborations among community-based programs and practitioners.
- Educate patients regarding the importance of public programs and dental health.
- Educate local, state, and federal policymakers on access to care issues.
- Become involved in discussions regarding public health infrastructure.
- Support research on oral health and disparities.
- Recruit individuals to join the oral healthcare workforce.
- Keep informed on care delivery systems, reimbursement schedules, and changes in public policy.
- Advocate improved funding and access for Medicaid recipients.
- Advocate better dental insurance and the inclusion of dental benefits in any new national health insurance plans.
- Advocate increased scope-of-practice regulations, or new workforce models, at the state or national level that would allow dental hygienists to provide more care to underserved patients in a variety of settings.

Dental therapy not only provides dental hygienists with an opportunity for career advancement but also for participating in a social good in addressing access to care and oral health disparities.

state. The practice of dental hygiene is regulated through each of these branches of state government. If left unregulated, the practice of dental hygiene could have the potential to harm patients. Dental hygiene is a highly skilled profession that requires professional education for the achievement and maintenance of competence. Government regulation is intended to minimize the public risk of untoward healthcare outcomes. The state dental practice act is the government regulation that most specifically controls the practice of dental hygiene.

Statutory Law

The legislative branch of government generally is responsible for the enactment of the state dental practice act, and state dental practice acts are overseen by state dental boards. The overall intent of state dental practice acts is to help ensure the protection of the public's health. In a limited number of states, the state constitution reserves for the people the right to enact laws independent of the legislature. For example, in the state of Washington, the constitution states,

> "the people enacted Initiative Measure No. 607, known as the Washington State Denturist Act, which established a program of licensure for denturists which provides a mechanism for consumer protection, and offers cost-effective alternatives for denture care services and products to individual consumers and the state" (WASH. REV. CODE §18.30.005 [2014]).

The state dental practice act may be a single law or a compilation of laws that regulate the practice of dentistry. These laws regulate the practice of dentistry by dentists, dental therapists, dental hygienists, denturists, dental assistants, expanded function dental auxiliary, and dental anesthesia assistants. Statutes that regulate the health professions are generally not all encompassing. In other words, dental hygienists must be familiar with the laws that deal specifically with dental hygiene as well as the general laws that protect the well-being of the state's citizens. For example, most states have enacted laws that require healthcare professionals to report suspected child abuse. This law may be found in acts that focus on child protection rather than on the practice of dental hygiene. Refer to the list that follows for a list of issues applicable to healthcare professionals that may be regulated by state law but may not be specifically incorporated into the state dental practice act.

ISSUES THAT MAY BE REGULATED BY STATE LAWS BUT MAY NOT BE SPECIFICALLY INCORPORATED INTO THE STATE DENTAL PRACTICE ACT

- Abuse reporting requirements (e.g., child, dependent adults, and domestic violence)
- Biomedical wastes and hazards management
- Business operation practices (e.g., rebating, credit agreements, business license, and advertising)
- Consent to treatment and informed consent
- Criminal activity
- Disability accommodation
- Education and training requirements (e.g., bloodborne pathogens)
- False healthcare claims
- Liability for volunteer services
- Malpractice or actions resulting from healthcare injuries
- Mandatory malpractice insurance
- Patient confidentiality and heightened protections (e.g., sexually transmitted diseases, mental health treatment, and substance abuse treatment)
- Public health reporting requirements (e.g., contagious or infectious diseases)

State Dental Boards

The governing bodies of dentistry may be referred to in terms such as Board of Dental Examiners, Board of Dentistry, State Dental Board, State Dental Commission, Dental Quality Assurance Commission, or Board of Dental Health Care. Dental hygiene representation in such regulatory bodies is common. For example, most dental boards are comprised of dentists, dental hygienists, and public members who are appointed by the governor of each state for specific terms. In Colorado, the dental board consists of seven dentist members, three dental hygienist members, and three members from the public at large. The governor appoints each member for a term of four years with a maximum of two consecutive terms (§12-220-105 [2021]). Alternatively, the practice of dental hygiene may be the purview of an elected regulatory body. In North Carolina, dental hygienists are elected to the

Board of Dental Examiners in an election as opposed to being appointed by the governor (§90-22 [1987]).

The job of members of state dental boards is to interpret and enforce the state dental practice acts, which are written by the state legislature. Generally, state dental boards do not have the power to change what is written in the state dental practice act without the state legislature passing an amendment. Additionally, as dentistry changes, state dental boards may interpret the state dental practice act to keep current with the profession, but they can only interpret this with what is written in the dental practice act. Along with interpreting and enforcing state dental practice acts, the functions of state dental boards may include the examination of dental hygienists for licensure; issuance, renewal, and revocation of dental hygiene licenses; investigation of disciplinary charges; and adoption of rules and regulations regarding the practice of dental hygiene. In some states, the regulatory body may be advised by a secondary body, which has

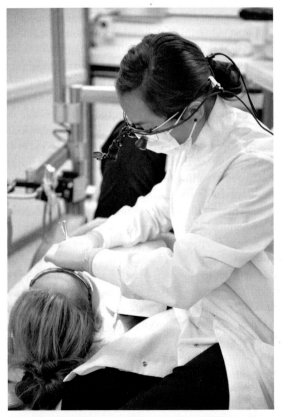

Courtesy: Idaho State University Department of Dental Hygiene.

greater dental hygiene representation, such as a council, as in Florida, or a Dental Hygienists Committee, as in New Mexico. The American Dental Hygienists' Association (ADHA) is a resource for information on states that utilize bodies secondary to dental boards.[1]

The Practice of Dental Hygiene

In the United States, the practice of dental hygiene is not nationally regulated. A movement towards an interstate licensure compact is being considered which would allow dental hygienists to work seamlessly within states that choose to join the compact. Until this becomes a reality, the practice of dental hygiene is different in each state. To obtain a dental hygiene license, applicants must take and pass a jurisprudence examination that delineates the laws and rules specific to the state's dental practice act. The professional obligation of dental hygienists is to be intimately familiar with the laws and regulations of the state in which they practice. A dental hygienist should, on an annual basis, review the applicable state dental practice act as laws and rules change to keep current with professional standards. A good time to do this may be at the time of license renewal, birth date, or another annually recurring date of significance. The contact information for the state licensing agency can be obtained from the American Association of Dental Boards at https://www.dentalboards.org.

State **statutory law** that regulates the practice of dental hygiene is likely to include provisions regarding the following: (1) licensure requirements, (2) licensure examination requirements, (3) licensure eligibility requirements, (4) licensure by endorsement, (5) approval of educational programs, (6) examination and disciplinary authority, (7) scope of practice, (8) supervision requirements, and (9) continuing education requirements. These laws provide a general outline of requirements, provisions, and limitations of the practice of dental hygiene and grant authority to the executive branch of government to implement administrative procedures and requirements.

Rules and Regulations

The executive branch of government is responsible for implementing the statutory law and providing more specific guidance and regulations regarding hygienist who does not pay the renewal registration fee forfeits their license. The board may reinstate the license without examination within 2 years of the date on which payment was due upon written application, proof of continued professional competence, and payment of all unpaid renewal and penalty fees (Alaska Statute Sec. 08.32.081[2022]).

If a dental hygienist does not renew their license but continues to practice, this constitutes practicing without a license and is a criminal offense. Depending upon the state and type of criminal offense, the violation may constitute a felony or a misdemeanor and is subject to disciplinary action. Dependent upon the violation, the penalty for noncompliance with licensure requirements may include a monetary fine and/ or imprisonment. In California, if a person is found guilty of a misdemeanor and convicted, they may be punished by imprisonment in a county jail of not less than 10 days nor more than 1 year, or by a fine of not less than one hundred dollars ($100) nor more than one thousand five hundred dollars ($1,500) (CAL. BUS. & PROF. CODE §1958 [2020]). In Connecticut, the fine cannot exceed five thousand dollars ($5,000) and the term served cannot be more than 5 years (CONN. GEN. STAT. §53a-41 [2014]).

Standards of Practice

Dental hygienists are obligated to comply with the accepted standards of professional practice and conduct. The standards may be specific to the practice of dental hygiene or more generally applicable to healthcare professionals. Dental hygienists are responsible for knowing the standards of practice in their state and ensuring that they are competent to engage in practice and comply with the provisions of their licensure. The standards of practice for dental hygiene are the minimum, competent, safe level of care provided by dental hygienists when they apply dental hygiene knowledge, skills, and attitudes to their practice. The ADHA published **Standards for Clinical Dental Hygiene Practice**, which can serve as a guideline for the most updated standards of practice.[2]

Some states have uniform standards of professional conduct for healthcare professionals, including the delineation of conduct and acts and conditions that constitute unprofessional conduct.

A dental hygiene license may be suspended or revoked on the basis of unprofessional conduct, violations of the laws and regulations governing the practice of dental hygiene, and clinical incompetence or the delivery of substandard care. *Unprofessional conduct* is a broad term that may encompass, but is not limited to, acts of fraud, misrepresentation, or deception; conviction of a felony; aiding and abetting, in the practice of dentistry or dental hygiene, any person not licensed to practice dentistry or dental hygiene; sexual conduct with a patient; and violation of state or federal laws. Dental hygienists also may have their practice restricted or suspended if they become impaired by reason of mental illness, physical illness, or habitual or excessive use or abuse of alcohol or controlled substances.

Continuing Education Requirements

Most states have continuing education requirements for maintaining a dental hygiene license. Such provisions may be found in state statutes or administrative rules, and they vary in the number of hours required to renew a license, the content of the course, and the course's presentation format. For example, in Ohio, every person licensed to practice as a dental hygienist and required to register with the state dental board must certify to the board at the time of applying for a renewal of registration in the two-year period preceding the registration period for which renewal is sought, the registrant completed a minimum of 24 hours of continuing dental hygiene education (Ohio 4715.25 [2021]).

Documentation or certification of compliance with continuing education requirements may be necessary when renewing the license. If documentation is not required at the time of license renewal, records of continuing education completion should be maintained for at least 2 bienniums as some states conduct random audits for compliance. In Ohio, "A licensed dental hygienist shall retain in the dental hygienist's records for a period of at least four years such receipts, vouchers, or certificates as may be necessary to document completion of continuing education programs. With cause, the board may request such documentation from licensed dental hygienists, and the board may request such documentation from licensed dental hygienists at random without cause" (Ohio 4714-25 ORC [2021]).

Licensing Fees

Initial licensure and renewal of the professional license require payment of a licensing fee. Dental hygienists who are not actively practicing dental hygiene and do not want to maintain a current license may be able to apply for an inactive license or retire their license. Although not all states have provisions for an inactive status, when available, an inactive or retired license may permit a dental hygienist to avoid the expense of maintaining an active license. It also permits the dental hygienist to maintain recognized professional status as a dental hygienist and to reactivate the license upon demonstration of professional competence (e.g., documentation of continuing education). Some states, such as Arkansas, require that a dental hygienist be practicing to maintain active licensure status. That law states, "Dental hygienists are automatically forfeited if they cease to practice either in the State of Arkansas or elsewhere for a period of two (2) years" (ARK. CODE ANN. §17-82-314 (a) [2015]).

Scope of Practice

The scope of dental hygiene practice varies among the states. The practice of dental hygiene includes educational, assessment, preventive, clinical, and other therapeutic services. The specific functions that can be legally performed in each of these aspects of dental hygiene practice are defined by state law. Examples of functions that are routinely allowed to be performed by the dental hygienist include the removal of deposits, accretions, and stains from the supragingival and subgingival surfaces of teeth by scaling, root planing, and polishing; the application of pit and fissure sealants, fluoride, and other topical therapeutic and preventive solutions; dental hygiene assessments and the charting of oral conditions; obtaining intraoral photographs; and exposing and interpreting oral radiographs. The practice of dental hygiene may include additional functions such as the administration of local anesthesia and nitrous oxide sedation as well as the performance of laser and restorative procedures. This expanded scope of practice typically requires approved instruction, formal endorsement, and/or heightened supervision. Regarding the administration of local anesthesia, in Ohio the law states that a dental hygienist may administer intraoral block and infiltration local anesthesia to a patient under *direct* supervision if the dental hygienist is in compliance with the education requirements and rules set forth by the dental board (Ohio 4715.230 ORC [2019]). Additionally, in Oregon, "Expanded Functions of Dental Hygienists must complete a course of instruction in a program accredited by the Commission on Dental Accreditation or other course of instruction approved by the Board" (Or. ADMIN. R. §818-035-0072 [2015]). General preclusions of dental hygiene practice include diagnosis for dental procedures or treatments and the cutting or removal of hard or soft tissues. The prescribing of drugs or medications is allowable in some states dependent upon the state's dental practice act. The ADHA provides a resource where the scope of practice for each state is presented.[3]

Dental hygienists have a legal and professional obligation to limit their practice to the scope of functions permitted by law in the jurisdiction in which they are practicing. If asked by an employing dentist or another licensed dental professional (e.g., dental therapist) to perform services that are clearly outside the legal scope of practice, the dental hygienist is obligated to decline to comply with the request. If it is unclear whether a procedure is within the legal scope of practice, the dental hygienist or employing dentist should seek clarification from the governing authority in the state of practice (e.g., board of dentistry or state dental board).

Supervision Requirements

The level of supervision required for the practice of dental hygiene varies by state, the scope of practice, and the location of the practice. Although the specific definitions for supervision are state specific, they can be generalized. **Direct supervision** generally requires a prior diagnosis of the patient's condition and authorization of a procedure by a dentist, the presence of a supervising dentist on the premises, and dentist approval of the work performed before patient dismissal. **Indirect supervision** requires a prior diagnosis of the patient's condition and authorization of a procedure by a dentist and the presence of a supervising dentist on the premises. **General supervision** requires that the services being delivered be authorized by the dentist along with other stipulations; however, the presence of the supervising dentist in the treatment facility is not required, but the dentist's availability for consultation may be required.

9

Dental Hygienist–Patient Relationship

PAMELA ZARKOWSKI AND MICHELE P. CARR

CHAPTER OUTLINE

LEARNING OUTCOMES

- Describe the professional obligation that exists between the dental hygienist and the patient.
- Recognize the difference between civil law and criminal law in the US legal system.
- Compare intentional torts and persons, intentional torts and property, and unintentional torts and negligence.
- List and evaluate the rights and responsibilities of the dental hygienist in the provider–patient relationship.
- State the patient's responsibilities when receiving oral health care.
- Describe the elements of informed consent.
- Define *malpractice* and *contributory negligence*.

The dental hygienist–patient relationship is a critical factor in the delivery of quality dental hygiene care. The dental hygienist–patient relationship is a two-party association that can only achieve its fullest potential with the committed participation of each of the parties. Patients enter into this therapeutic relationship with certain expectations. Dental hygienists must understand these expectations through communication with their patients. Suppose dental hygienists are unable to meet their patients' expressed expectations. In that case, the patients must understand this limitation and either accept the limitation and alter their expectations or seek care from an alternative provider who is able to meet the expectations. The dental hygienist has a professional obligation in this relationship to comply with the laws that govern the practice of dental hygiene and to deliver oral healthcare services that meet the standards of care of the profession. Failure to fulfill this professional obligation can result in untoward consequences to the patient and

Intentional Torts to Property

The physical invasion of intruding on land without authorization is a form of intentional tort. Interference with the possession of an individual's property is another form of intentional tort. For example, finding a colleague's lost handpiece and keeping it as one's own property is interference.

Unintentional Tort of Negligence

Negligence is an unintentional tort that involves the failure to act as a reasonable, prudent person under similar circumstances. Malpractice is a form of negligence that, in the context of medicine and dentistry, includes all liability-producing conduct resulting from the delivery of healthcare services.

Rights and Responsibilities of the Dental Hygienist and Patient

The dental hygienist–patient relationship includes a number of rights and responsibilities for both parties (Boxes 9.1 and 9.2). Failure by either party to meet its obligations can result in litigation. Dental hygienists must become familiar with their responsibilities to patients, which include the following:

> **• BOX 9.1** **The Dental Hygienist's Responsibilities When Delivering Oral Health Care**
>
> - Possess a proper license and registration, comply with all laws, and practice within the scope of practice as dictated by state law.
> - Exercise reasonable skill, care, and judgment in the assessment, diagnosis, and treatment of patients.
> - Use standard drugs, materials, and techniques.
> - Complete treatment within a reasonable time.
> - Charge reasonable fees.
> - Never abandon a patient and always arrange for care during an absence.
> - Refer unusual cases to a specialist.
> - Maintain patient privacy and confidentiality.
> - Keep accurate records.
> - Give adequate instructions to the patient.
> - Maintain a level of knowledge and practice within the code of ethics.

> **• BOX 9.2** **The Patient's Responsibilities When Receiving Oral Health Care**
>
> - Pay a reasonable fee in a reasonable time.
> - Cooperate in care and keep appointments.
> - Provide accurate answers about dental or medical history and current health status.
> - Follow instructions, including home care instruction.

- Dental hygienists must have a current license for the state in which they practice and have it displayed as required. An individual who fails to renew a license or who is denied a license cannot practice. Dental hygienists must perform only the legally allowed duties with appropriate supervision.
- Dental hygienists must deliver care that meets the standard of a reasonable person in the profession. A reasonable person is one who would use suitable judgment based on the circumstances. A practitioner makes a judgment or decision based on his or her educational training and experience. A dental hygienist is held to the standard of a dental hygienist, not a dentist or a physician.
- A dental hygienist must use medications, materials, and techniques recognized by the profession. Patients trust that the dental hygienist will recommend or use therapeutic treatments recognized by professional groups, such as the American Dental Association (ADA) or the American Academy of Periodontology (AAP).
- An office must complete treatment in a timely manner. An office that chooses to delay or extend treatment for any reason, such as in the case of a patient with a difficult personality, is at risk of extending treatment beyond an acceptable time.
- An office should charge fees that are usual, customary, and reasonable.
- An office cannot stop the treatment of a patient if harm will occur. The discontinuation of the provider–patient relationship requires appropriate notification to avoid **abandonment**. The necessary notification includes informing the patient in writing, allowing emergency care to be provided for a specific period, suggesting that the patient seek another provider, and providing the patient

with an opportunity to obtain a copy of their dental records. An office also must have a policy for short-term absence. To meet this obligation, a dental office may use an answering service, voice mail, or pagers to allow for emergency contact.

- A dental hygienist has a duty to understand their abilities and limitations and to collaborate with the dentist to appropriately refer to other providers.
- A dental hygienist must respect a patient's right to privacy. A patient's privacy is protected by specific laws such as the Health Insurance Portability and Accountability Act (HIPAA). Patient information cannot be shared with unauthorized parties without the patient's permission. Office staff must be careful not to divulge information without a patient's consent. Office staff must be cautious not to have casual or public conversations about a patient that would violate the patient's privacy and must never post patient information on social media.
- An office is required to record information received in a logical, complete, and accurate manner. Records may include written documentation (e.g., collected data, diagnoses, treatment plans, and a description of the treatment provided), radiographs, images, and models. Patients have the right to obtain a copy of their records. State regulations may outline fees to obtain medical and dental records.
- An office must give the patient appropriate and understandable pretreatment and posttreatment instructions. Instructions may be provided verbally and in writing. In offices with diverse patient populations, instructions should be available in commonly spoken languages to facilitate understanding. Translation services are also available.
- Dental hygienists are required to remain current with all aspects of patient care. It is important to attend continuing education courses, read scientific literature, and use other educational sources to keep knowledge and skill levels up to date. In addition, an awareness of and adherence to a professional code of ethics are imperative.

Patients seek care, trusting that their legal rights will not be violated and that their health and oral health status will not be harmed. When harm or injury does occur, several remedies may be available through the judicial system.

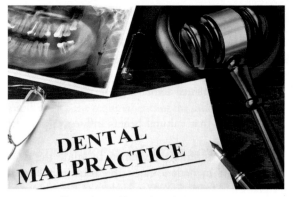

From: https://www.istockphoto.com.

Legal Actions for Healthcare Injuries

When the care delivered by a dental hygienist results in injury, the injured patient may seek compensation and justice through the courts. The three most common actions relating to health care are (1) failure to obtain informed consent, (2) professional malpractice, and (3) breach of contract. At the core of each of these actions is the question of whether the dental hygienist violated a duty owed to the patient. The American Dental Hygienists' Association (ADHA) recognizes that the dental hygienist has the following professional responsibilities to patients[*]:

- Provide oral health care utilizing high levels of professional knowledge, judgment, and skill.
- Maintain a work environment that minimizes the risk of harm.
- Serve all [patients] without discrimination, and avoid action toward any individual or group that may be interpreted as discriminatory.
- Hold professional [patient] relationships confidential.
- Communicate with [patients] in a respectful manner.
- Promote ethical behavior and high standards of care by all dental hygienists.
- Serve as an advocate for the welfare of [patients].
- Provide [patients] with the information necessary to make informed decisions about their oral health,

---

[*]Excerpted from: American Dental Hygienists' Association. *Code of Ethics for Dental Hygienists, Chicago*; 2019. The use of the term *client* in the code has been replaced with *patient*.

that they have been informed of their condition and consent to the plan of care. For high-risk procedures, such as surgery, the use of a comprehensive and individualized consent form is advisable.

Informed Refusal

Patients may refuse recommended treatment or referrals. They may refuse radiographs, anesthesia for a root planing and scaling treatment, or a referral to a periodontist. Patient refusals must be documented in the patient record. This protects the provider if there is future litigation because there is a record of a provider and patient interaction. The informed refusal process parallels the informed consent process. The patient must be informed of the procedure or recommendation. The reason and need for the procedure must be clearly explained. The oral and general health risks should be described. For example, a patient refusing to agree to radiographs must be informed that a lack of radiographs will limit the dental hygienist's ability to evaluate periodontal status, bone loss, and other oral health conditions. The dental hygienist can also educate the patient about the relationship between oral and systemic health conditions that may be impacted by less-than-ideal oral health care. An informed refusal, sometimes referred to as a declination of treatment, should be documented. It is important to get the patient's signature and signatures from a provider and a witness. It is advisable not to allow patients to consistently refuse recommended treatment. An office policy should be determined concerning patients who refuse recommended treatment as it may be putting the dental hygienist and dentist at risk for allegations of malpractice. Appropriate patient termination policies should be developed.

Professional Malpractice

Professional malpractice had its beginning in common law, as did informed consent. However, many jurisdictions have codified the requirements of claims relating to health care.

Malpractice Defined

In general, dental **malpractice** is the failure of an oral healthcare provider to exercise the degree of care, skill, and learning expected of a reasonably prudent oral healthcare provider, in the class to which he or she belongs within the state, acting in the same or similar circumstances. Some states provide protection against malpractice actions to providers delivering care as volunteers and not for compensation.

Malpractice may be established when a provider is found to have violated the standard of care. The standard of care can be established legislatively, administratively, and through expert testimony.

Dental hygienists violate the standard of care when they injure a patient by not using the care, knowledge, skill, and ability possessed by other dental hygienists. For example, a dental hygienist would violate the standard of care if they failed to obtain a comprehensive health history on a patient before performing periodontal therapy. The dental hygienist may commit malpractice if this violation of the standard of care results in injury to the patient. For example, if a patient has a heart condition that requires antibiotic premedication and the dental hygienist performs periodontal therapy without knowing this condition, the dental hygienist may commit malpractice if the patient develops bacterial endocarditis. The standard of care for dental hygiene includes responsibilities in patient assessment, treatment planning, patient education, treatment, and evaluation.

Shared Responsibility

Healthcare injuries result from both the provider's failure to meet the standard of care and the patient's failure to comply with the treatment plan. In such situations, the responsibility for the injury is shared by the patient and recognized as **contributory negligence**. Responsibility for healthcare injuries also may be shared between the provider and employer. The legal doctrine of *respondeat superior* stands for the proposition that employers act through their employees or agents and are therefore responsible for the negligent acts of their employees or agents. As licensed professionals, a dental hygienist and dentist may be *jointly* named in a lawsuit alleging malpractice.

Statute of Limitations

A **statute of limitations** is a statutory provision that limits the period within which an injured party can file a legal action. The purpose of these time limitations is to protect against stale claims that will be difficult to judge because of limited documentation and undependable recollection of events. Statutes of limitations for healthcare injury or malpractice actions vary by state; however, they usually are in the range of 2 to 4 years from the date of the alleged act, omission, neglect, or occurrence. Given that some injuries are not known at the time of their occurrence, a statute of limitations also provides for a period (1 to 2 years) for filing an action after the discovery of an injury. For injuries to minors, the statute of limitations is tolled until they reach the age of majority:

• A statute of limitation is the time allowed to file a court case. Statutes of limitation apply in both civil and criminal cases. The statute of limitations for some cases is as short as six months, while some serious criminal offenses have no limit and can be filed at any time, even decades after the crime occurred. Most statutes of limitation range from one to eight years.[2]

Reporting Requirements

Some states, such as Arizona and Oklahoma, require that malpractice settlements and judgments against dental hygienists be reported to the state health profession regulatory board. Such notice may then serve as a cause for an investigation by the regulatory board regarding the professional's practice. In addition to state requirements, the National Practitioner Data Bank is a national program that collects and discloses negative information on healthcare practitioners, including malpractice awards and loss of a license (https://www.npdb.hrsa.gov).

Breach of Contract

The most common **breach of contract** claim associated with healthcare injuries is that the healthcare provider promised the patient that the injury suffered would not occur. For example, statements indicating that a proposed procedure will take care of "someone's troubles" and that there is "nothing much to the procedure" may represent promises that cannot be kept. Healthcare providers are not expected to be guarantors of healthcare outcomes. Therefore, the dental hygienist should be careful not to make statements that a patient may interpret as a guarantee of outcome.

Summary

This chapter provides a general overview of the legal context of the dental hygienist–patient relationship. The dental hygienist–patient relationship is a two-sided relationship with rights and responsibilities on each side. As a healthcare professional, the dental hygienist has an ethical and legal obligation to uphold the standards of the profession and avoid injury to the patient. When injury that should have been avoided does occur, the legal system is designed to provide retribution and compensation to the patient and society. Dental hygienists are responsible for understanding their legal obligations and are encouraged to seek legal counsel when specific issues of concern arise.

PRACTICE POINTER

During a recall appointment, the dental hygienist spends more time with the patient than the dentist and other office personnel do, and as such relationships are built. It is helpful to get acquainted with and learn facts about patients to discuss at future appointments. Showing interest in patients as individuals can be beneficial for the practice and in turn, can play a role in the patient's decision to accept recommended treatment and to return for recurring appointments.

respect, dignity, and professionalism. Dental hygienists, together with the practices in which they are employed, will prosper when recognized for their professional contributions and acknowledged as valued members of a team. Compliance with federal and state employment laws is one way for an employer to give dental hygienists the professional recognition they deserve.

Although an employer should be familiar with and comply with legal employment obligations, uninformed and unintentional violations can occur. Questions, potential oversights, and unintended violations should be brought to the employer's attention for resolution. However, when this does not result in a satisfactory resolution and a dental hygienist suspects that their employment rights have been violated, an attorney or appropriate agency should be contacted for guidance and possible legal resolution. Such action should be viewed as the ethical and professional obligation of a dental hygienist.

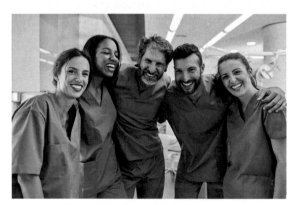

From: https://www.istockphoto.com.

Seeking and Obtaining Employment

When seeking employment, a dental hygienist may explore several different forums. Dental hygienist positions frequently are announced in classified advertisements in local newspapers and professional publications, such as newsletters and journals. Dental hygienist job placement services, which may be advertised in professional newsletters or online, are another source for identifying available positions. Examples include professional Facebook groups, LinkedIn, and Monster.com. Word of mouth and networking with fellow professionals at meetings, continuing education programs, and community service events also can be valuable mechanisms for finding well-suited employment opportunities. Formal job announcements generally indicate the application procedure and provide details regarding the preferred mode of contact (telephone, email, or in person) and résumé submission.

The selection process generally includes an interview with the employer. The interview may be limited to a review of the résumé and job description followed by a question-and-answer period between the interviewer and the dental hygienist. In some situations, it may include a working interview, which provides an opportunity for the employer to assess the applicant's professional competence. A working interview provides an opportunity for the licensed dental hygienist to assess the office environment, including scheduling, record-keeping practices, disinfection and sterilization protocols, and other aspects of the business. A dental hygienist should be paid for a working interview to comply with labor laws. Frequently the employer or staff will meet with the dental hygienist to provide feedback. However, it is important to recognize that this is not a one-sided event and that the dental hygienist should be assessing whether or not they are satisfied with the office climate and delivery of oral healthcare services.

When preparing for an interview, the dental hygienist should consider the following strategies:

- Prepare a concise, accurate, and professional résumé that highlights the educational background, employment history, licensure, and professional experiences, such as association membership, presentations, and honors.
- Obtain a job description and develop questions concerning practice philosophies and protocols, referral strategies, documentation guidelines, performance evaluation, and other pertinent information.
- Anticipate questions and plan responses to inquiries about career goals, professional skills and judgment, commitment to lifelong learning, and potential contributions to the practice.
- Be familiar with proper and improper employment inquiries during the interview process.

Limitations exist regarding the questions that may legally be asked during the hiring process. The following list provides examples of *permissible* inquiries during the application and interview process:

- Full name and any different names necessary to verify employment history

- Date of birth
- Length of residency in a particular state or city
- Name of relatives already employed by the employer
- Ability to perform the duties of the position with or without accommodation
- Ability to meet specified work schedules and attendance requirements
- Legal eligibility to work in the United States
- Languages that can be spoken and written fluently
- Education and employment history
- Criminal conviction history
- Emergency contact

The application and interview process is intended to support the selection of an applicant who can perform the functions of the available position. Questions are classified as *impermissible* when the information sought could be used in a discriminatory manner and is irrelevant to assessing an applicant's qualifications for a position. However, once a hiring decision is made, certain additional information may be necessary for personnel records and employee benefit programs. The following list provides examples of inquiries *not* permitted during the application or interview process:

- Age, only if the candidate is 18 or older
- Original name when changed by court order or marriage
- Marital and family status or related questions
- Number of children and their ages or related questions
- Sex orientation or gender identity
- National origin, ancestry, or descent
- Religion or creed
- Race or color
- Height and weight
- Disability status
- Arrest record
- Required list of affiliations and memberships
- Garnishment of wages
- Native language

During the application and interview process, applicants should be cautious not to offer information voluntarily that cannot be solicited legally by the employer. Although a dental hygienist who is the proud parent of two fabulous children might be inclined to comment on the children after noticing pictures of the employer's children, the dental hygienist should think twice about doing that. A discussion of children could raise concerns about child care arrangements and a sick child's impact on the employee's attendance record. Personal information can be shared following the hiring decision.

> ### PRACTICE POINTER
>
> Employees should use caution in sharing personal information at work that could influence an employer's attitude about the employee and potentially be used for discriminatory reasons.

Employment Relationship

There are two general **employment categories**: (1) at will and (2) term. The *at-will* category is best described as employment with an indefinite duration. This means that the employment relationship can be terminated at the will of either the employer or employee for any or no reason with or without an explanation or warning. A dentist can inform a dental hygienist at the end of a workday that his or her employment in the office is terminated, effective immediately. Termination decisions customarily are accompanied by notice (e.g., 2 weeks before the end of the employment relationship) or severance pay. However, the termination of an at-will employment relationship can legally occur without notice, severance pay, or a statement of cause as long the decision was not made for a discriminatory or retaliatory reason. In an at-will situation, an employee can resign at any time.

The category *term* is best described as employment with a definite duration. For example, a dental hygienist may sign an employment contract for 12 months. An employment contract generally has language that specifies the conditions under which the employment relationship can be terminated before the completion of the duration. The legal term for these conditions is *just cause* or *good cause. Cause* is reasonable job-related grounds for dismissal based on, for example, failure to satisfactorily perform job duties. The employment relationship cannot be terminated without breaching the contract unless just cause exists, which is a specified (i.e., contractually agreed upon) and nondiscriminatory reason for termination. Some states have wrongful discharge protections which specifically state that an employee can only be terminated for good cause.

experienced a violation of their employment rights may file a charge of discrimination with the EEOC. The process is not complicated; however, specific guidelines and time frames must be followed (see the box on this page). It is unlawful for an employer to retaliate or take adverse action (e.g., by refusing to hire, denying job benefits, or making threats) against an employee who opposes any violations of the employment discrimination laws (e.g., refuses to answer impermissible interview questions, suggests treatment is unequal based on disability, or complains to a coworker about sexually harassing behavior) or files a complaint with the EEOC (42 U.S.C. §2000e-30). More details about the federal laws prohibiting employment discrimination can be obtained at the EEOC website (https://www.eeoc.gov).

Individuals also may file complaints with their state commission (e.g., human rights commission or civil rights office) when concern exists that state laws are being violated.

Other Laws Providing Employee Protections

Family Medical Leave Act of 1993

The Family Medical Leave Act of 1993 (FMLA), 29 U.S.C. §§2601–2654, is a federal law that makes available medically necessary leave to qualified employees. This act was created to balance the demands of the workplace with the needs of families, to promote the stability and economic security of families, and to promote national interests in preserving family integrity.

The FMLA applies to public and private employers with 50 or more employees. To be eligible, an employee must have worked for the employer for 12 months and worked at least 1250 hours over the previous 12 months. Under the FMLA an employer must grant an eligible employee up to 12 weeks of unpaid leave during a 12-month period for the following reasons:

- Birth and care of a newborn child within 1 year of birth
- Placement of a child for adoption or foster care
- Provision of care for an immediate family member (spouse, child, or parent) with a serious health condition (includes in *loco parentis*)

FILING AN EEOC CLAIM FOR DISCRIMINATION

- Any individual who believes that their employment rights have been violated may file a charge of discrimination with the EEOC.
  A charge may be filed personally or by mail to the nearest EEOC office. An individual can identify the closest EEOC office by contacting the EEOC at 800-669-4000 or 800-669-6820 (TTY), or ASL Video Phone 844-224-5122, or by using the EEOC Field Office List at https://www.eeoc.gov/field-office.
- The following information should be available when filing a complaint: (1) the name, address, and telephone number of the person being treated unfairly, (2) the name, address, and telephone number of the employer or agency alleged to have discriminated and the number of employees at the workplace, (3) a brief description of the event or events that are unfair or harassing, and (4) the dates of the event(s).
- Strict time limits exist within which charges must be filed. A charge must be filed with the EEOC within 180 days from the date of the alleged violation. Exceptions exist, but contacting the EEOC promptly when discrimination is suspected is best.
- Once a charge has been filed, the employer is notified. Resolution of the charges is determined based on a review of the facts by the EEOC.
- Resolution of the charge may involve various courses of action. An attempt may be made to remedy the discrimination. Remedies may include, but are not limited to, back pay, promotion, reinstatement, hiring, front pay, reasonable accommodation, or other actions that would make the complainant "whole." If the EEOC's attempt to conciliate a remedy is unsuccessful, legal action may be available.
- EEOC services are free.
- Additional information may be obtained from the US Equal Employment Opportunity Commission at 131 M Street NE, Washington, DC 20507; 202-663-4900 or 202-633-4494 (TTY) or eeoc.gov
  Publications are available that advise employees of their equal opportunity employment rights. To obtain this information, contact the EEOC at eeoc.gov/eeoc-publications.

- Serious health condition that makes an employee unable to perform the function of their position
- Any qualifying exigency arising out of the fact that a family member (spouse, son or daughter, or par-

ent) is a covered military member on "covered active duty"

- 26 workweeks of leave during a single 12-month period to care for a covered service member with a serious injury or illness if the eligible employee is the service member's spouse, son, daughter, parent, or next of kin (military caregiver leave)

In some circumstances, the FMLA permits leave to be taken intermittently, such as taking leave in blocks of time or reducing a regular daily or weekly schedule. When possible, employees should give their employer 30 days of notice before beginning an FMLA leave. During an approved FMLA leave, an employer must maintain the insurance benefits provided as a part of the employment relationship. Upon return to employment, an employee is required to be restored to their original position or to an equivalent position with equivalent pay, benefits, and other terms and conditions of employment. More details on the FMLA can be obtained at the US Department of Labor website.

States have passed bills related to paid and unpaid family and medical leave. The bills fall into three main categories: Family Medical Leave; states that only have pregnancy leave statutes; and since 2020, specific pandemic and COVID-19 statutes (https://www.ncsl.org/research/labor-and-employment/state-family-and-medical-leave-laws.aspx). States may enact laws that extend the provisions of the FMLA—for example, domestic violence leave is available in the state of Washington for victims of domestic violence, sexual assault, and stalking to seek legal or law enforcement assistance; to seek treatment by a healthcare provider for physical or mental injuries; to obtain services from a domestic violence shelter, rape crisis center, or other social services; or to participate in safety planning activities (Domestic Violence Leave, ch. 49.76 WASH. REV. CODE).

Occupational Safety and Health Act of 1970

The Occupational Safety and Health Act (OSHA) of 1970, 29 U.S.C. §§651-678, is a federal law intended to ensure working conditions free from recognized hazards to the safety and health of employees. The law places responsibility on employers and employees to comply with established standards and

training requirements intended to minimize the number of personal injuries and illnesses that arise out of employment. In general, employers are obligated to provide employment free from recognized hazards that may cause serious physical harm to their employees. For example, OSHA standards require that the employer provide personal protective equipment (PPE) in the dental office to minimize the hazards associated with contact with bloodborne and airborne pathogens. The US Department of Labor updates the OSHA guidelines. During 2020 and the COVID-19 pandemic, OSHA provided information specific to Dentistry Workers and Employers. It included information about recommended PPE ensembles for dentistry related to specific procedures and cleaning and disinfection (https://www.osha.gov/coronavirus/control-prevention/dentistry). Unlike the Centers for Disease Control and Prevention (CDC) recommendations which are advisory, OSHA guidance includes references to mandatory requirements under the OSHA guidelines. Employees, in turn, are obligated to comply with OSHA standards applicable to their scope of employment. State laws also may be enacted that equal or exceed the requirements imposed by OSHA. More details on OSHA can be obtained at the OSHA website (http://www.osha.gov).

State workers' compensation provisions provide relief for injured employees while acting in the course of their employment. Dental hygienists who are injured at work should notify their employer of the injury and seek assistance in complying with the workers' compensation program's requirements. The home pages of all of the state government websites can be found at https://www.usa.gov/agencies.

Sexual Harassment

Like many employment settings, the dental office environment provides opportunities for frequent interaction among colleagues. Multiple levels of interactions occur, including employer–employee, employee–employee, and employer/employee–patient/client. Each of these levels of interaction provides an opportunity for inappropriate behavior.

Oral healthcare providers work in close contact with their colleagues and patients. Dental hygienists

Summary

Because of the importance of commerce in society, employment is highly regulated by federal and state laws and statutes. Such regulation is intended to protect the welfare of society by safeguarding the individual interests of employees. Dental hygienists are likely to work as employees during the course of their career. They must be informed of federal and state employment laws and act to ensure that their rights are upheld.

REFERENCE

1. Zarkowski P. Sexual harassment: it's unacceptable, *J Mass Dent Society* 67(3), 20–23, 2018.

Simulations and Applications

Healthy People 2030 oral health objectives, and he further offered to have her come and visit sometime to learn more about the type of care he is providing. He also explained the legality of his ability to provide care within the dental hygiene scope of care in schools and other locations due to the practice act in Wisconsin. Mario also used this interaction as an opportunity to ask Dr. Brooks if he could refer patients with Medicaid insurance to her office since he struggles with finding them restorative dental care when he identifies possible areas of concern. Dr. Brooks also noted that she has concerns with taxpayer dollars being used to help children who do not take the responsibility to maintain good oral health. Lastly, Mario tried to share the current evidence-based practices regarding when and when not to seal a tooth. Dr. Brooks abruptly ended the conversation, and Mario put his phone down and walked down the hall of the school to get his next patient from their classroom.

Questions

1. Does Mario have a right to include this child in his school-based sealant program if he is a patient of record in Dr. Brooks' office?
2. Following his assessment, is Mario able to diagnose the need for dental sealants?
3. According to the CDC recommendations for school-based sealant programs, should Mario have placed a sealant on a tooth that has a noncavitated carious lesion? Discuss your answer using the CDC guidelines.
4. List and discuss the Healthy People 2030 oral health objectives that school-based sealant programs address.
5. List and describe which core values from the ADHA Code of Ethics for Dental Hygienists relate to this school-based sealant program.
6. What do you think about Dr. Brooks' comment about personal responsibility and taxpayer dollars being used to provide care to this population?
7. How would you have handled this situation if you were Mario?

CASE 2

To Sell or Not to Sell

Carla Loiacono
Concorde College, Texas

Dr. Chris Hunt has been in private practice for 10 years in a suburb of a large metroplex. Dr. Hunt graduated from an Advanced Education in General Dentistry (AEGD) program and associated with a large general practice for 3 years before buying a building and opening a solo practice. Although all phases of general dentistry are performed, the focus of the practice is moving toward adult esthetic dentistry. Ms. Lisa Meyer is a dental hygienist who has been in Dr. Hunt's practice full-time for 3 years and enjoys a great relationship with her patients and an active schedule. Ms. Meyer has been a full-time practitioner for 6 years, and this is the second office in which she has worked. Her greatest professional rewards are the trust that has developed between her and her patients and the improvement she has seen in their oral health.

Dr. Hunt recently completed a continuing education series on esthetic dentistry and hired a practice management company to review the office. The course director and the management team both stressed the importance of using the hygienist to "sell dentistry" to patients. The course and the management team both identified certain phrases and inferences hygienists should use to help the patient make the "right" choice.

Dr. Hunt approaches Ms. Meyer and explains her new role to her. Ms. Meyer is uncomfortable with this change in her job duties because she feels that she would be using her professional position to possibly unduly influence patients toward making certain treatment choices. "Am I taking advantage of the trust that I worked hard to establish with our patients?" she asks. "No," Dr. Hunt replies. "Actually, you are educating our patients about the benefits of the highest-quality care. In fact, to make this arrangement more attractive I am including an incentive plan with cash bonuses for every case that you sell." This statement concerns Ms. Meyer because she feels that these incentives may eventually place her own economic self-interest in conflict with the patient's best interest.

Questions

1. What aspects of informed consent are important to this case?
2. What are the dental hygienist's obligations to the patient in this situation?
3. List and discuss the core values expressed in the ADHA Code of Ethics for Dental Hygienists that are related to this case.
4. What are the possible legal issues related to this case?
5. Using the ethical decision-making model, analyze this case.

Patients with Special Needs

Michele P. Carr
The Ohio State University

Nancy has been working for the past year as a dental hygienist in a very busy ambulatory healthcare facility that treats persons who have intellectual and developmental disabilities. The majority of patients treated at this facility are covered under government assistance plans, and when procedures are not covered by the insurance plan, the facility writes off the charge for the services. After working in this setting, Nancy found that generally the patient's oral hygiene was poor regardless of their ability to perform oral hygiene procedures on their own or if the patient was dependent upon a caregiver. In spite of having dedicated numerous hours training caregivers and providing oral hygiene instruction to the patients, Nancy has met with little success regarding the improvement of oral hygiene and periodontal health in patients.

Recently Nancy implemented a program in which patients who are periodontally involved or continuously have poor oral hygiene return for 3-month re-care visits instead of the typical 6-month visits. This approach worked in her previous private practice office and had positive results. However, in this new facility, she is not seeing any improvement in oral health and questions the value, time, and cost to treat these patients when the facility is not being compensated and she sees no benefit to the patient. Many patients are waiting months to get a dental hygiene appointment and eliminating nonresponsive patients on 3-month re-care visits would allow for more appointments, to be available for those who are waiting. Nancy is frustrated and wonders how to balance dental needs and economics with this patient population.

Questions

1. List and discuss the core values from the ADHA Code of Ethics for Dental Hygienists related to this case.
2. What are the possible legal principles related to this case?
3. Using the ethical decision-making model, analyze this case.

CASE 6

Standard Precautions

Donna Wittmayer
Clark College, Washington

A dental hygiene student was assigned to a community outreach site where dental care was provided to underserved populations. One morning, as she was reviewing the charts of the patients she would be treating that day, she noted that one of the patients was HIV-positive and had a history of hepatitis C. The student understood the principles of, and always practiced, standard precaution procedures; thus, she was not concerned about treating the patient. Before this patient's appointment time, the dental assistant at the site approached the dental hygiene student and directed her to their supply of disposable laboratory coats. The assistant stated, "You should wear one of these when treating this patient, so your cloth laboratory coat will not become contaminated." She also instructed the student to place contaminated instruments in a special container of disinfecting solution after she had completed treatment on the patient. After the contaminated instruments had soaked for 30 minutes, they would be processed through the ultrasonic bath and then would be run through the autoclave twice to guarantee the instruments were completely sterilized.

Questions

1. Should the student follow the recommended procedures at the extramural site, or should she follow the accepted standard procedures? What are the alternatives for the student?
2. List and discuss the core values from the ADHA Code of Ethics for Dental Hygienists related to this case.
3. Using the ADHA Standards of Professional Responsibility, discuss the responsibilities of the dental hygienist that are applicable to this case.
4. What are the possible legal issues related to this case?
5. Using the ethical decision-making model, analyze this case.

CASE 7

Warming Up

Gary Chiodo
University of Washington School of Dentistry

A recently graduated dental hygienist has taken a position in a group practice periodontal office. The professional staff in this office includes four periodontists and six dental hygienists. Although she has been on the job only 3 months, the dental hygienist is truly enjoying the advanced level of practice involved in caring for the patients. Patients referred into this specialty practice are in need of various types of periodontal therapy, and the periodontists maximize the dental hygienists' talents in performing nonsurgical interventions. This dental hygienist has observed the degree of care and thoroughness demonstrated by the periodontists and other hygienists, and she respects their abilities and level of professionalism.

For the past few weeks, however, she has been bothered by one of the periodontists who seems to frequently make inappropriate comments about her appearance, tease her about private body parts, tell her sexually oriented jokes, and constantly ask her to go out on a date with him. Lately, this doctor has begun giving her neck and shoulder massages in the employee breakroom if he finds her there alone. She has asked him to stop because these actions make her uncomfortable and has politely explained that she is not interested in dating him. These protests have not deterred the amorous advances of this dentist who is recently divorced and very vocal about being "in the marketplace."

Today, while the dental hygienist is in her operatory sharpening instruments, the dentist comes in and begins rubbing her neck and shoulders. She rises from her chair and asks him to please stop and to confine his future interactions with her to professional issues. The dentist becomes upset at this rejection and says, "You know, I control a significant part of your salary. I don't see why you are always brushing me aside. You'd be lucky to have someone like me. Maybe you should think more about your future here and warm up a little."

Questions

1. List and discuss the core values from the ADHA Code of Ethics for Dental Hygienists related to this case.
2. Using the ADHA Standards of Professional Responsibility, discuss the responsibilities of the dental hygienist that are applicable to this case.
3. What are the possible legal issues related to this case? Specifically, what does Title VII of the Civil Rights Act state related to sexual harassment?
4. Using the ethical decision-making model, analyze this case.
5. How might the dental hygienist deal with this situation so as not to create animosity between her and others in the office? Should she be concerned about creating animosity?

CASE 8

Patient Confession

Debi Gerger
West Coast University, California

A 35-year-old female comes to your office as a regular 6-month recall patient. She has been a patient in the practice since it opened 7 years ago and is always faithful in coming to her appointments. In general, she is in good health. The dentist completed one bridge a couple of years ago, and her probing depths are usually generalized 3 mm to 4 mm with light supragingival and subgingival calculus localized to the lower anterior teeth. Some marginal gingival inflammation is present from poor brushing technique.

This patient has been seen by the same dentist for years. The practice is building, and with four dental hygienists now employed, patients are often scheduled with the first available dental hygienist. This patient has been seen by a different dental hygienist and then returns to the dental hygienist who normally sees her each recall. After the medical history review, the dental hygienist proceeds to do a full mouth probing and discovers that today's readings are significantly lower than the last visit and compliments the patient on her great improvements.

The patient then reveals that the last dental hygienist told her that her pockets were so bad that if she did not brush and floss better she would lose all her teeth. She was also told that her cleaning needed to be done every 4 months to help control the "mess she was in." The patient said she was taking this information in, even though it was delivered in a demeaning manner by this other dental hygienist while she was being "tortured by the scaling procedure." She was in pain not only during the visit but for 3 days afterward. The patient also said her 16-year-old daughter had a cleaning by the same person and was in tears from the pain when she came home. The daughter's chart was pulled, and "good oral hygiene and light plaque" was noted. This is not the first time you have heard this kind of information about this dental hygienist.

Questions

1. List and discuss the core values from the ADHA Code of Ethics for Dental Hygienists related to this case.
2. Using the ADHA Standards of Professional Responsibility, discuss the responsibilities of the dental hygienist that are applicable to this case.
3. What are the possible legal issues related to this case?
4. Using the ethical decision-making model, analyze this case.
5. How would you handle this situation?
6. Would you recommend to the patient that she call the state dental board?
7. Would you tell the patient that you have heard these kinds of comments before?
8. Would you say something to the dentist?
9. Would you talk with the other dental hygienist?

Guidelines or Mandates?

Shavonne R. Healy

The World Health Organization (WHO) officially declared an outbreak of severe acute respiratory syndrome (SARS-CoV-2) a global pandemic in 2019. To help reduce the spread of a highly infectious respiratory disease and to preserve personal protective equipment (PPE) for first responders, the Occupational Safety and Health Administration (OSHA) and the Centers for Disease Control and Prevention (CDC) recommended that all elective medical and dental procedures be postponed. State governors across the United States began issuing stay-at-home orders that corresponded with WHO, OSHA, and CDC recommendations to temporarily suspend elective and nonemergency dental procedures until further notice. OSHA and the CDC released interim guidelines for dental professionals to refrain from aerosol-generating procedures to prevent the risk of healthcare-associated SARS-CoV-2 transmission. The American Dental Hygienists' Association (ADHA) publishes interim guidance on returning to work that was aligned with OSHA and the CDC. The media reported that the virus was and remains a highly contagious, aerosol-transmissible disease with high morbidity and mortality rates.

Claire is a 36-year-old mother of two young children. She works as a solo dental hygiene practitioner for a busy periodontal office. Her employer, a dentist, has informed her that the office will resume business effective immediately, including nonemergency procedures, without the use of aerosol-generating devices in *hygiene* operatories. The number of deaths has increased, and little is known yet about the safety and efficacy of working during a pandemic.

Claire has been monitoring the ongoing guidance from regulatory and public health agencies and discusses with the dentist the recommendations from the WHO, OSHA, CDC, and ADHA to postpone nonemergency procedures until further notice. Claire also asks the dentist if the practice has secured the recommended PPE, physical barriers, air-handling system, and supplies for patient triage protocols. The dentist reacts angrily and tells Claire that those are "guidelines," not mandates, and that the office will be proceeding as it had prior to the start of the pandemic. The dentist lets Claire know she is expected to return to work along with the rest of the staff.

Questions

1. List and discuss the core values from the ADHA Code of Ethics for Dental Hygienists related to this case.
2. Using the ADHA Standards of Professional Responsibility, discuss the responsibilities of the dental hygienist that are applicable to this case.
3. What are the possible legal issues related to this case?
4. What are the possible implications for the practice and licensed providers if contact tracing from a patient who contracted the virus identifies the practice as the source and the evidence-based CDC Infection Prevention and Control in Dental Settings recommendations, which include the interim guidelines related to this virus, were not followed?
5. If Claire has further questions related to the return to work for nonemergency treatment procedures, who can she contact?
6. Using the ethical decision-making model, analyze this case.

CASE 10

Misdiagnosis

Laura Fassacesia
Plaza College Dental Hygiene Program

Andrew Dean is a 58-year-old male, who is an accountant in New York City. Andrew's dentist is Dr. Howard Daviss. Dr. Daviss has treated Andrew for the past 25 years, they are golf buddies, and Andrew trusts Dr. Daviss. Dr. Daviss's office is in the building where Andrew works, and it is very convenient for him.

Andrew's wife, Razia, sees different dentist who referred her to a specialist, Dr. Fornix, a periodontist. Razia thinks it is a good idea for Andrew to see the periodontist for a evaluation. Andrew asked Dr. Daviss and the dental hygienist at his office for a referral to a periodontist, but Andrew was told "You do not need to see a periodontitis—you have gingivitis only, which does not warrant a referral."

A few months later, on a Saturday, Andrew began to have a toothache. When he was brushing his teeth he felt pain. When he looked in the mirror, he noticed the gingiva around his lower right molar was swollen and bleeding. He called Dr. Daviss, who put him on an antibiotic. Dr. Daviss was away for the weekend, but he explained to Andrew that he may have an infection and need root canal therapy. Dr. Daviss expected the pain to improve after 24 hours of the antibiotic. The pain did not improve, so Andrew made an emergency appointment to see his wife's periodontist, Dr. Fornix. The periodontist took a periapical x-ray of #30 and a cone beam CT scan. Tooth #30 had an infection and a class II furcation visible on the x-rays. Dr. Fornix did emergency surgery, but he could not save the tooth. The x-rays and subsequent surgery showed approximately 75% bone loss at the site. Less than the apical third of the root was embedded in bone. Dr. Fornix asked Andrew to get his last set of x-rays and his last perio chart from his dentist for review at his post-op visit. Andrew went home and was very upset.

On Monday, Andrew called Dr. Daviss's office to request his records. The last x-rays, a set of four horizontal bitewings, had been taken 2 years ago. The only full periodontal charting had been completed 25 years ago, at his initial appointment. The last updates had

been recorded 3 years ago. The updates included recession on teeth #24 and #25, a 5-mm pocket on #3-MB, and a 4-mm pocket on #14-DL with bleeding. There was no mention of pocketing, bone loss, or furcation involvement on #30. When Dr. Fornix called Dr. Daviss, Dr. Daviss said his dental hygienist had written, "Patient had gingivitis and need to improve his homecare, 6-month recalls" in the chart. They never graded or staged his periodontal disease with the 2017 American Academy of Periodontology (AAP) Classifications.

Dr. Fornix invited Andrew to come to his office for a periodontal evaluation as a new patient. The dental hygienist at Dr. Fornix's office took a full mouth series of x-rays (FMX) and recorded a comprehensive periodontal chart including:

- Probing depths
- Gingival margin
- Mucogingival junction
- Clinical attachment level (CAL)
- Mobility
- Furcations recorded with a Nabers probe
- Bleeding upon probing
- Suppuration

The hygienist also recorded: radiography bone loss (RBL), plaque, and calculus levels.

When all of the recordings were completed, the patient was staged and graded according to the AAP 2017 Classifications.

The comprehensive exam is part 0 of the five phases of dental treatment. Andrew was misdiagnosed by Dr. Daviss office, he does not have gingivitis; he has active periodontitis with no records indicating when periodontitis began.

Andrew's periodontal diagnosis was generalized Stage III, Grade B: mucogingival deformities. Andrew's treatment plan is as follows:

- phase 0 was accomplished at the first visit of assessment;
- phase I, 6 sextants of scaling and root planing with a 4- to 6-week reevaluation;

CASE 12

The Dental Therapist

Anne High
Rochester Community and Technical College, Minnesota

Molly is a dental hygienist employed as a dental therapist (DT) in a state that requires this provider to have dual licensure as a DT and a dental hygienist in order to provide care to underserved populations in public health settings. A DT practices under the general supervision of a licensed dentist in the state and is able to perform simple extractions, restore teeth, perform some pulp therapies, and write prescriptions for a limited range of drugs in addition to the full dental hygiene scope of practice. A formal collaborative agreement between the dentist and DT has to be on record with the state board of dentistry. The dentist has to be involved in the dental diagnosis and treatment planning for all patients.

Under normal circumstances, Molly uses the rural dental clinic's telehealth capabilities and communicated with the dentist via live video conference. This arrangement allows the dentist to assist in diagnosis and treatment planning for patients with restorative or surgical needs. Most of the patients Molly treats are young children with dental decay, and often a variety of procedures are required while treating the teeth. The treatment plans often include antibiotic regimens, pulp therapy, stainless-steel crowns, restorations, and extraction of primary teeth.

On one particular Thursday, Molly was practicing in the rural clinic and received an emergency phone call from the mother of a patient of record. The patient had not completed his treatment plan last summer and was now in acute pain. Although the dentist had helped plan the treatment for the patient 9 months ago, the tooth indicated for a restoration now presented with an infected pulp. Molly had often treated cases similar to this one and knew what the dentist would probably recommend, but he was out of town and unable to be reached for consultation. Because Molly did not want the child to lose the tooth, she went ahead and treated the patient without consulting the dentist.

Questions

1. List and discuss the core values from the ADHA Code of Ethics for Dental Hygienists related to this case.
2. Using the ADHA Standards of Professional Responsibility, discuss the responsibilities of the dental hygienist that are applicable to this case.
3. What are the possible legal issues related to this case?
4. Using the ethical decision-making model, analyze this case.

CASE 13

Summer Employment

Stephanie Bossenberger
Weber State University, Utah

Mary Ann Fisher has been a dental assistant at Dr. Martan's office for the past 5 years. She functions as a chairside dental assistant, exposing radiographs as directed, and acting as the infection control officer for the dental office. During this time, Mary Ann has been pursuing her education to become a dental hygienist and recently completed her first year of the program. She has been an above-average student both academically and clinically. However, she has stated that she does not understand why becoming a dental hygienist takes so long. Several times during clinic, Mary Ann has been cited by faculty for taking shortcuts and avoiding evaluations. Since being counseled on this behavior, she has been more careful to follow protocol. Her clinical performance is at an acceptable level for a student completing the first year of instruction.

School ended in mid-May, and Mary Ann was able to resume her employment full-time in Dr. Martan's office. Dr. Martan is very proud of Mary Ann and often boasts to patients of her accomplishments and that she will be a dental hygienist very soon. Mary Ann continued with the work she had done in the office for a year, polishing each patient's teeth before the dentist's examination. Now that she has become more adept at instrumentation, she has probed and scaled the teeth of several patients when she has considered it necessary.

Mia, the part-time dental hygienist in the office, knew that Mary Ann was stretching her dental assisting duties and, after careful consideration, decided it was time to have a meeting to talk about what was going on in the office. At the meeting, Mia gave out copies of the state Dental Practice Act, and everyone understood the reason for the clarification of duties.

The dentist thanked Mia and said he thought it was "very informative and interesting." For the next 6 weeks, Mary Ann was careful to only provide services that were listed in the Dental Practice Act, but after that she was scaling and probing teeth again.

Mia was disappointed in the dentist and the dental assistant as she thought they would adhere to the legal scope of practice after their meeting. Although Mia was a bit anxious about being fired, she was quite sure that Dr. Martan would understand her concern for the patients in his practice and not wish them to receive substandard care. The more she thought about the situation, the angrier she became. She realized that she is required to report to the Board of Dental Practice any infraction of the state Dental Practice Act.

Questions

1. Should Mia call the dental hygiene program faculty?
2. Is Mia required to tell Dr. Martan that she is going to report this infraction to the state dental board before she does?
3. List and discuss the core values from the ADHA Code of Ethics for Dental Hygienists related to this case.
4. Using the ADHA Standards of Professional Responsibility, discuss the responsibilities of the dental hygienist that are applicable to this case.
5. What are the possible legal issues related to this case?
6. Using the ethical decision-making model, analyze this case.

CASE 16

Systemic Racism

Alexandra D.E. Sheppard
University of Alberta, Canada

Ashley is a registered dental hygienist in a midsize city. Ashley just started working in a general dental practice 3 weeks ago and was especially happy to obtain the position, as the office is located close to home. Ashley shadowed the dentist and the previous dental hygienist during the final year of dental hygiene studies and has dreamed of working in this office. For the past 2 years, a pandemic has affected all aspects of life from attending school and small business closures to restrictions on gatherings, to a concern about the attainment of appropriate personal protective equipment (PPE) for dental practices.

Ashley reviews the schedule for the day. The sterilization technician looks at the schedule as well and says loudly, "Why are they coming in? I do not like these people at all, as they are the cause of the virus and the death of my grandmother. Personally, I think you need to do an extra-thorough disinfection of the operatory after they leave. I will double-sterilize the instruments so the next patient does not get ill from their germs. Make sure you wear an N95 mask. I really dislike these people." The dental assistant nods in agreement and both walk out of the sterilization area. Ashley looks down and becomes quiet.

Ashley is of Asian ancestry. Throughout the day, the comments from the sterilization tech and the affirmation from the dental assistant have been bothering Ashley. That evening Ashley decides to use the six-step decision-making model to help address this ethical situation.

Questions

1. List and discuss the core values from the ADHA Code of Ethics for Dental Hygienists related to this case.
2. Using the ADHA Standards of Professional Responsibility, discuss the responsibilities of the dental hygienist that are applicable to this case.
3. What are the possible legal issues related to this case?
4. Using the ethical decision-making model, analyze this case.
5. Discuss the pros and cons of each option that Ashley could consider as part of coming to a decision.
6. What are the professional responsibilities and considerations that Ashley should consider?

CASE 17

The Maxillary Bridge

Mary Turner
Sacramento City College, California

Dr. Agar, my dentist employer, has the Timothy family—father, mother, and two daughters—as patients. The family is a struggling, lower-middle-class family trying to pay for their daughters' college educations. The family had recently received from Mr. Timothy's employer a family health policy with dental coverage. Before receiving this coverage, paying for dental care was always a substantial problem for the Timothy family. Unfortunately, Mr. Timothy lost his job 2 weeks ago and is now looking for other employment.

At this time, Mr. Timothy is in the middle of several appointments for periodontal debridement before the placement of a new maxillary anterior bridge. Mr. Timothy has asked Dr. Agar to postdate an insurance claim form so that his treatment is covered by the dental plan. Because Dr. Agar would like to help his patient, he has asked me to alter the dates of the dental hygiene services that I will be providing to Mr. Timothy so they can also be included on the claim form.

Mr. Timothy needs the treatment, especially because he is looking for new employment. I know the family well as one of the daughters used to babysit my daughter—they need whatever benefits the insurance will pay.

Questions

1. Should I comply with Dr. Agar's wishes? After all, he is my boss.
2. List and discuss the core values from the ADHA Code of Ethics for Dental Hygienists related to this case.
3. What are the possible legal issues related to this case?
4. Using the ethical decision-making model, analyze this case.

Fitting In

Pamela Overman
University of Missouri-Kansas City

Sarah is happy to have a job as a dental hygienist for Dr. Stanley Dard. Sarah is a newly divorced mother of two teenagers and has to stay in this area as a part of the divorce settlement. Dr. Dard is a member of the state dental board, and he really values the periodontal aspect of care. He serves as a state clinical examiner, and he checks patients very meticulously to make sure everyone receives the best of care. Recently, Sarah has seen a side of Dr. Dard that has her concerned. She walked by his operatory as he was presenting a proposed treatment plan to a new patient. The patient was a devout Muslim woman, wearing a traditional loose-fitting dress and a scarf covering her hair. When discussing the fees with the patient, Dr. Dard quoted fees that were considerably higher than those he typically presented. Sarah assumed she had misheard until it happened again. This second time it was a Hispanic man, who has limited English-speaking skills. She waits for an opportune moment and asked Dr. Dard about how he sets fees for services when presenting treatment plans. He said he sets fees based on the difficulty of the treatment and seemed disinclined to go into much more depth.

Today, Sara sees a treatment plan presentation on Dr. Dard's schedule, and the treatment room door is closed when she walks by. After the final patient of the day, Dr. Dard asks Sarah to stop by his office for a discussion about her performance in his office. He is not sure she is fitting in. Sarah is panicked and not sure what to do next.

Questions

1. What action, if any, should Sarah take immediately?
2. List and discuss the core values from the ADHA Code of Ethics for Dental Hygienists related to this case.
3. What are the possible legal issues related to this case?
4. How might Dr. Dard view this situation?
5. Is there some way Sarah could have avoided being placed in this situation?
6. Using the ethical decision-making model, analyze this case.

CASE 24
New Skills

Ann McCann
Texas A&M University

The ability to treat children was the reason that Harper Mallone, RDH, went to dental hygiene school. She loved working at the office of Dr. Marvin Stallsworth because it was a family practice and she had the opportunity to treat many children. She hoped to have her own children someday—caring for them was her special love, and she was good at it.

Dr. Stallsworth believed in saving as much tooth structure as possible and often did sealants on teeth with small occlusal carious lesions. This procedure (called an enameloplasty) involved excavating only the carious enamel tissue in the pits and fissures of the tooth with a small bur and then placing a sealant in the area. Harper would identify the carious lesions during her oral examination at patient recall appointments. When Dr. Stallsworth came into the dental hygiene operatory for his examination of the patient, he would prepare the tooth and then have Harper place the sealant.

One morning, Dr. Stallsworth requested that Harper learn how to do an enameloplasty so that she could perform the entire sealant procedure herself. He said it was very easy to do, and it would free him up to spend more time with his restorative patients. This would be a win-win situation for both the office and the patient by decreasing the length of the dental hygiene appointment. When the next patient arrived who needed a sealant, Dr. Stallsworth showed Harper how to do the enameloplasty and had her use a high-speed handpiece to remove the carious enamel. Harper found the procedure fairly easy and was looking forward to performing the procedure on future patients.

She enthusiastically described her new skill to a fellow dental hygienist at the monthly dental hygiene society meeting. Her friend expressed surprise that she was placing sealant restorations and told her she should not be restoring teeth. Harper did not know what to do. Her employer wanted her to do the procedure independently, and she liked having more responsibility at the office.

Questions

1. Would this procedure be legal in some states or regions?
2. Whose responsibility is it to know if this task is within the dental hygiene scope of practice for Harper's state?
3. List and discuss the core values from the ADHA Code of Ethics for Dental Hygienists related to this case.
4. Using the ADHA Standards of Professional Responsibility, discuss the responsibilities of the dental hygienist that are applicable to this case.
5. What are the possible legal issues related to this case?
6. Using the ethical decision-making model, analyze this case.

CASE 27

Breach of Contract?

Shavonne R. Healy

Dr. Patty Jones is a well-known and highly respected periodontist in the area. Her current hygienist of 10 years is leaving the practice, and Jack, a highly skilled and experienced dental hygienist, was referred for the position by a trusted colleague. During the interviewing process, Jack informed the doctor of his *terms and conditions* and asked that they be documented in his employment agreement. He understood that the previous hygienist worked 8- to 9-hour days Tuesday to Thursday with a 30-minute lunch break and all day on Friday with no lunch break. Jack informed Dr. Jones that he would need an hour for lunch if considered for the position.

Jack also shared his concern about the 60-minute time frame being allotted for periodontal therapy and voiced that he would need additional time with patients involving more than one quadrant of scaling and root planing. Dr. Jones agreed to Jack's requests, and they signed the employment agreement. Jack returned the next week to begin his new role as a periodontal therapist at Dr. Jones's office.

Jack had been working for Dr. Jones for 3 months when he started to notice changes in his schedule. He saw that his lunch hour had been reduced to 30 minutes and that patients needing four quadrants of periodontal therapy were being scheduled for 60-minute appointments. When Jack approached the office manager about the unannounced changes to his schedule, she responded, "Dr. Jones wanted hygiene to go back to the regular schedule. It's how we are used to doing it, and the old hygienist never complained about the way we do things."

Questions

1. Is the employment agreement between Jack and Dr. Jones a valid contract?
2. What are the possible legal implications of the employment agreement being breached?
3. Should Jack provide Dr. Jones with an opportunity to remedy the situation?
4. What would you do if you were Jack?

CASE 28

The Dentist Dental Assistant

Monica L. Hospenthal
Pierce College Fort Steilacoom, Washington

Shari is a dental hygienist who has worked for the past 3 years at Dr. Merriweather's practice. Recently she was faced with a highly illegal and unethical situation when her dentist was out of the country on vacation.

Dr. Merriweather is a family-friendly employer, fosters a positive environment, provides benefits, and most importantly, practices quality and ethical dentistry. He also allows his staff to work to their full scope of practice within the law.

Dr. Merriweather sometimes takes 4 week breaks and closes the practice. He is an avid bicyclist and had been planning for months to leave on a Saturday morning for a 4-week bike tour in Spain. Shari often schedules to take temporary assignments for part of these 4-week breaks.

Shari realized on a Saturday afternoon that she had forgotten her loupes and face shield in her operatory room. Because she and all the employees have an office key, she decided to swing by the office on Sunday to collect her things for her Monday temping position.

As she drove into the parking lot of the building, she noticed Katrina's car in the parking lot. Katrina is a newer expanded functions dental assistant (EFDA) with the practice but has been a dental assistant (DA) for over 10 years. She recently went back to school to become an EFDA, and therefore, Dr. Merriweather recently promoted her to lead DA.

Shari enters through the back door of the office and greets a cheerful hello to Katrina to let her know who it is. As Shari walks around the corner, she sees Katrina working on a patient! There is a full restorative cassette open and a local anesthetic syringe, which clearly has already been used. The patient has a rubber dam on #6 through #11, and Katrina is holding a high-speed hand-piece, looking as if she is getting ready to use it. Katrina looks at Shari and says, "Oh, hi! I was just placing a filling for my friend because she doesn't have the money to go to the dentist. It was just a small chip." Katrina turns back to the patient to continue the treatment.

Katrina is allowed to place and finish restorations in the state. However, dental assistants are not educated or allowed by law to perform local anesthetic or prepare teeth.

Questions

1. List and discuss the core values from the ADHA Code of Ethics for Dental Hygienists related to this case.
2. Using the ADHA Standards of Professional Responsibility, discuss the responsibilities of the dental hygienist that are applicable to this case.
3. What are the possible legal issues related to this case?
4. Looking at the events through Dr. Merriweather's eyes, how might he view the situation?
5. Using the ethical decision-making model, analyze this case.

CASE 29

Agnes Day

Phyllis L. Beemsterboer
Center for Ethics in Health Care
Oregon Health and Science University

Background

Agnes Day has lived in her own home, alone with her cat, since her husband died 6 years ago. She is 83 years old, very independent, and very private. Her independence and privacy have been challenged for the past several months, however, after she suffered a stroke with hemiparesis on the left side. Her left hand is badly contracted and has little feeling. She drags her left foot when she walks. She occasionally falls but can walk about her home, though she refuses to use a cane. She can no longer drive and has recently started paying a young couple to drive her for errands such as grocery shopping and going to the doctor. Her son and daughter both live in the area and help her around the house. She will go out for meals with them and allow them to bring in meals and have family gatherings at the house, but she will not let them go to doctor visits with her "because she does not want them to take over." Similarly, she has never mentioned the falls to them (or to anyone else), fearing that if her children knew about them they would try to force her to live with them or, worse, in a nursing home options she loathes. Her other medical problems include diabetes, for which she takes insulin, and chronic congestive heart failure, for which she takes furosemide (a diuretic).

A Medical Crisis

A few weeks ago Ms. Day suffered a cut on her left hand. Because she has little feeling in the hand, the cut did not hurt, and Ms. Day felt no reason to seek medical care. Over the next few days, the cut became infected, and the infection spread all the way to her shoulder. Her entire arm became swollen and red. She had fever and chills, and she became confused and short of breath. When her son dropped by for a visit and saw how ill she was, he immediately called 911. Ms. Day was admitted to the hospital.

In the Hospital

Over During the 10 days in the hospital, Ms. Day received IV antibiotics, drainage of her wound, and management of her diabetes and congestive heart failure. As she returned to eating solid food, she bit a nut and cracked a tooth, but the tooth does not hurt, and Ms. Day is now eager to be discharged. However, Ms. Day's son and daughter insist that it is not safe to send their mother home. Their mother's recent bouts of confusion have made them very doubtful about her *capacity* to manage on her own at home, especially given her physical limitations. Ms. Day, on the other hand, is very clear with everyone that she is going back home. She has agreed to have a visiting nurse come to the house to pack her wounds but will not allow anyone to stay at the house. She has also agreed, with some evident impatience and irritation, to make an appointment to see her dentist. Her children insist on a psychiatric consult to evaluate Ms. Day's decision-making capacity. When the psychiatrists report that they believe Ms. Day has the capacity to make the decision to go home, the children ask that several members of the team caring for their mother (Ms. Day's primary nurse, attending physician, social worker, and physical therapist) meet with them for a care conference. Ms. Day's daughter speaks first: "Mother might have fooled that psychiatrist, but we have seen how confused she gets sometimes, and now that she's so weak after being in the hospital—how can we just send her back to that house by herself?"

Back Home

Ms. Day goes home. The plan is for a visiting home health nurse to see her daily to pack the wound. She will continue with oral antibiotics. The young couple will continue to run errands, and her son and daughter plan to bring meals more often. The RN care manager in the office of Ms. Day's primary care physician (PCP) will

CASE 30

Cyberbullying

Toni M. Roucka
Marquette University School of Dentistry

Julia, a bright 13-year-old, had been a patient of Dr. Bill Moyer for most of her life. She always had very good oral hygiene and was fortunate to never have needed a dental restoration. As a result, when Julia came for dental visits it was Joy, Dr. Moyer's hygienist, with whom Julia spent the most time.

The last two times Julia had come in for her routine dental care, Joy had noticed a stark change in Julia's behavior. She seemed quieter, and her oral hygiene was lacking. In fact, her overall personal hygiene seemed to be suffering. Previously very talkative and animated, Julia barely answered Joy's questions regarding her teeth.

At first, Joy attributed Julia's behavior to "teenage growing pains." Most adolescents seem to go through a phase like this at some point. Because Joy had developed a rapport with Julia over the years, she felt comfortable and compelled to ask her how things were going in her life. What was new? What was the "teenage buzz" around town? What was the latest "technology" taking the teen world by storm? Maybe she could get to the root of what seemed to be bothering her. That got a rise out of Julia. She snapped back stating, "There is *no* buzz or great new technology as far as I am concerned. I am sick of people on social media spreading lies and rumors about me. I might as well *never* go on the Internet again!" Further questioning revealed that Julia was a victim of cyberbullying and her parents did not know about it. Joy did not know exactly what to do next. Dr. Moyer was in surgery, and she could not interrupt him to ask. Joy decided to speak with Julia's mother right after the appointment to alert her to the problem. Though annoyed at first, Julia seemed to be grateful that the truth was finally revealed. She was tired of pretending everything was okay in her life.

Questions

1. Did Joy do the right thing by talking to Julia's mother about their conversation?
2. Should Joy have gotten Dr. Moyer's opinion about the situation first?
3. List and discuss the core values from the ADHA Code of Ethics for Dental Hygienists related to this case.
4. Using the ADHA Standards of Professional Responsibility, discuss the responsibilities of the dental hygienist that are applicable to this case.
5. Should cyberbullying be considered a form of "child abuse" and thus rise to the level of mandatory reporting to child protective services?
6. Could Julia have handled the situation differently? If so, how?

SUGGESTED ACTIVITIES

The following activities can be used to enhance the study of ethics and law in dental hygiene. These activities can be accomplished individually or in small working groups.

1. Review the ADHA Standards of Clinical Dental Hygiene Practice and review the six standards to formulate risk management strategies for clinical practice.
2. Explore the medical and nursing literature on bioethics to see the range of references available.
3. Look at a medical textbook on ethics. Compare the types of issues that are presented and discussed to those presented and discussed in this textbook.
4. What types of ethical dilemmas are on the news or being discussed in social media?
5. List how many articles in the media, over a period of time, relate to ethical issues. What principle is most often cited?
6. Search the web and list the number of sites that refer to dental health care and ethics.
7. Pick one of the following topics and research the issue as it affects health care and healthcare delivery:
   - Abortion
   - Access to care
   - Assisted suicide/Death with dignity
   - Blood transfusion
   - Clinical and translational research
   - Emergency care
   - Health maintenance organizations
   - Informed consent
   - Law and life support
   - Paternalism
   - Transplantation
   - End-of-life care
   - Integrative medicine
   - Harvesting reproductive cells
8. Locate the code of ethics from a healthcare professional group, such as physical therapists, chiropractors, or medical technologists. Compare with the ADHA Code.
9. Locate the code of ethics for another medical organization, such as the American Medical Association (AMA) or American Nurses Association (ANA). Compare it with the ADHA Code and/or the ADA Code.
10. Access the website for the American Society for Dental Ethics, and explore what the group does.
11. Access the websites for the following centers for ethical study and research the materials available:
   - Hastings Center, Garrison, NY
   - Center for Health Care Ethics, St. Louis, MO
   - Center for Ethics in Health Care, Portland, OR
   - Midwest Bioethics Center, Kansas City, MO
   - Ethics Institute of Dartmouth College, Hanover, NH
   - Kennedy Institute of Ethics, Washington, DC
   - Mayo Clinic Biomedical Ethics Program, Rochester, MN
12. Research and list the ethical issues that can arise in relation to dental research.
13. Establish small study groups to explore different cultures and then compare and contrast common beliefs and practices.
14. Discuss ethnocentrism and how it can affect the practice of dental hygiene and dentistry.
15. Look up the following ethics and legal words and use them in a sentence:
   - Louche
   - Probity
   - Turpitude
   - Peccant
   - Malversation
   - Malfeasance
   - Canard
   - Perfidy
   - Phronesis
   - Iniquitous
16. Establish small groups, and research the state dental practice acts from several different regions in the United States, then compare results.
17. Research a recent dental malpractice case in your state or region, then identify the risk manage-

ment errors that may have led to the legal action and suggest risk management solutions.

18. Analyze the risk management practices in the clinical setting in which you are working or plan to work.

19. Research the issues surrounding the professional with drug or alcohol impairment, and determine how those issues are handled in your state or region, both ethically and legally.

20. Access your state government website, and find out the rights and responsibilities of employers and employees.

TESTLETS

Testlet 1

Charlee is a dental hygienist in a busy practice with three dentists, one other hygienist, and six dental assistants. The office also supports an administrative staff of four. Oak Grove Dentistry is a high-volume practice, with 250 to 300 patient visits per week among clinical practitioners. New patients to the practice are seen first by the dental hygienists, who take the medical history and perform the initial examination, including the current periodontal status and restorative needs.

Although Charlee is impressed by the quality of services that the patients receive, she is distressed by what she believes is a wide disparity between her clinical assessment of restorative need and that of one of the dentists who finds many more carious lesions than she notes. Her observations were confirmed when she discussed the issue with the other hygienist and one of the dentists, both of whom expressed similar concerns.

When Charlee approached Dr. Kane, the owner of the practice, with her concern, she was told clearly that a definitive diagnosis of caries and oral disease is within the scope of practice for the dentist, not the dental hygienist. When Charlee added that the other dental hygienist also was concerned, Dr. Kane intimated that she was a "troublemaker" and any further allegations that he was not acting in the best interests of his patients would not be tolerated.

1. This case presents issues that may be
   a. unethical
   b. illegal
   c. grounds for malpractice
   d. all of the above
   e. none of the above

2. The *main* principle involved in this case is
   a. autonomy
   b. beneficence
   c. nonmaleficence
   d. justice
   e. veracity

3. Does Charlee have any responsibility to the patients in this practice?
   a. No; she is an employee, not the owner, of the practice.
   b. Yes; she must adhere to the ADHA Code of Ethics.

4. What section of the ADHA Code of Ethics "Standards" applies to this situation?
   a. "To ourselves as professionals"
   b. "To clients"
   c. "To employees and employers"
   d. "To the dental hygiene profession"
   e. "To the community and society"

Testlet 2

A patient assigned to Callie Rose in the periodontal practice at which she works has a severe case of periodontal disease, Stage IV, Grade C. The dentist's employer initially examined the patient and, because of the amount of calculus present, sent her for scaling and debridement. The patient is elderly, somewhat shy, and keeps saying that she wants Callie to do "whatever is necessary" so she can keep her teeth. Callie is concerned that the patient does not fully understand her disease, the scope and expense of treatment, and treatment options.

1. What healthcare obligation is most important in this case?
   a. Confidentiality
   b. Informed consent
   c. Paternalism
   d. Veracity

2. Making sure the patient understands the course of treatment is honoring the ethical principle of
   a. autonomy
   b. beneficence
   c. justice
   d. nonmaleficence
   e. veracity

3. Callie should be concerned about this situation because the patient is
   a. elderly and shy
   b. too trusting
   c. yet to be diagnosed by the dentist
   d. not well informed about her oral health

4. What section of the ADHA Code of Ethics "Standards" applies to this situation?
   a. "To ourselves as professionals."
   b. "To clients."
   c. "To employees and employers."
   d. "To the dental hygiene profession."
   e. "To the community and society."

Testlet 3

A new patient, Marissa, is a 15-year-old who is seeing a dental hygienist for dental care for the first time. In this practice, radiographs are taken of every new patient as part of the diagnostic data gathering. As a safety precaution before taking radiographs, females potentially of childbearing age are asked whether they could be pregnant. Marissa, aware that her mother is in the waiting room, very quietly tells the hygienist that she is pregnant. She also says that her parents are unaware of her condition and begs the hygienist not to tell her mother or the dentist.

1. Which *main* ethical principles are involved for the dental hygienist in this case?
   a. Autonomy and nonmaleficence.
   b. Beneficence and justice.
   c. Nonmaleficence and veracity.
   d. Justice and autonomy.
   e. All of the above.

2. At what age would this person become an adult?
   a. When she turns 16 years of age.
   b. When she turns 18 years of age.
   c. When she pays for her own dental care.
   d. When the state law says she is an adult.

3. Taking radiographs of pregnant women is not recommended because
   a. radiation is dangerous for a fetus
   b. radiation may be dangerous for a fetus
   c. pregnancy gingivitis is a risk
   d. of concerns for the health of the mother

4. The dental hygienist should first
   a. try to convince Marissa to discuss her pregnancy with her mother
   b. inform the dentist of this dilemma
   c. contact Marissa's mother and inform her of the pregnancy
   d. delay dental hygiene treatment

Testlet 4

Julie is a part-time dental assistant and a graduate of an accredited dental assisting program. She was credentialed by the state to expose radiographs and place pit and fissure sealants as expanded functions dental auxiliary (EFDA). She works in a practice the 2 days of the week that the dental hygienist is not scheduled and generally sees a full client load. Many of her clients were children when she began her employment, but lately, she has noticed that many of them are now adults on Medicaid.

The dentist explained to her that he would scale the client's teeth and directed Julie to polish them because that is "as good as the hygienist would be able to do." When Julie checked the Medicaid claim form for these clients, she found that her services were being billed as "adult prophylaxis." This is not in her scope of practice as an EFDA.

The dentist's employer told Julie that the Medicaid reimbursement rates were so poor that he believed these clients were getting more than adequate treatment. He pointed out that he was one of the few dentists in the area who provided any treatment to Medicaid patients and that Julie should be happy to assist in this valuable service.

1. This case presents issues that are
   a. unethical
   b. illegal
   c. grounds for malpractice
   d. all of the above
   e. none of the above

2. Which ethical principle is most important in this case?
   a. Autonomy.
   b. Beneficence.
   c. Nonmaleficence.
   d. Justice.
   e. Veracity.

3. The clinical function of polishing teeth
   a. is a traditional dental assisting duty
   b. is an expanded dental assisting duty
   c. is a function of the dental hygienist
   d. can be delegated by the dentist
   e. depends on state law

Testlet 5

Renee is happily employed in a large suburban practice that sees mostly families and children. A number of hygienists work full-time, and a few come in for only a day or two. Getting to know all of them has been fun, and they cover for each other when they have to attend a child's school play or sporting event. Jessie is a hygienist with whom Renee has developed a growing friendship, and they often have lunch together.

One very busy day, Renee is scheduled to complete treatment on a rather complicated periodontal case when Jessie asks her to switch patients. The office follows a policy of continuity of care, and each hygienist completes his or her own patients. Renee asks why, and her friend indicates that she does not want to provide dental hygiene treatment to the patient as she is part of a "same-sex couple" and that this is not what her church believes in.

1. This case presents issues that may be
   a. unfriendly
   b. illegal
   c. grounds for malpractice
   d. all of the above
   e. none of the above

2. The main ethical principle raised in this case is
   a. autonomy
   b. paternalism
   c. nonmaleficence
   d. justice
   e. veracity

3. Which of the following would be appropriate for Renee to do in this situation?
   a. Refer Jessie to the office manager with her request.
   b. Refer Jessie to the practice's policies and procedures manual.
   c. Tell Jessie no and discuss with her the legal implications of her request.
   d. All of the above.
   e. None of the above.

Testlet 6

Karen is a dental hygienist in the practice of Joe Alvins, DDS. Stacy is treating Ms. Holloway, a patient with acute gingivitis, who is also seeing a naturopathic physician to help her with her allergies.

Ms. Holloway has three large posterior amalgam alloys that she insisted needed to be replaced with the composite because her naturopath told her "mercury fillings" were unhealthy. Dr. Alvins has told her that in most cases alloy has proven to be a better choice in posterior teeth, but Ms. Holloway has made it pretty clear that she was going to do what her naturopath told her to do. Dr. Alvins has tried to help her understand the procedure, risks associated, and material science of both restorations. After a long-informed consent discussion and process, Dr. Alvins was treatment planning the composites but not very happy about it. He knew it was not the best option for the patient.

Dr. Alvins was frustrated that his professional skills and judgment had been undermined by another clinician. He asked Karen to tell the patient that the naturopath was making a diagnosis out of his field of expertise and to talk the patient into adhering to his treatment plan.

1. Which of the following principles and values are most involved in this case?
   a. Autonomy and informed consent.
   b. Confidentiality and justice.
   c. Trust and veracity.
   d. Paternalism and beneficence.

2. This case presents issues that may be
   a. unethical
   b. illegal
   c. grounds for malpractice
   d. all of the above
   e. none of the above

3. The dental hygienist should follow the dentist's request because
   a. the dentist is the ultimately responsible individual
   b. evidence-based dentistry does not support this treatment option
   c. she is an employee of the practice
   d. all of the above

Testlet 7

Each dental hygiene and dental student in the Greenfield University Dental School is assigned to an off-campus rotation at a rural clinical site for a 4-week period, living in housing provided by the local community. Although the clinical experience is fantastic, the students are finding the quieter lifestyle boring.

On social media, several students have commented about the lack of things to do while on this rotation and made fun of what the locals do for fun, calling local dances and events "white trash diversions." One hygiene student, Laurel, is upset about this and talks to several of her colleagues about this

lack of professionalism. She is met with a resounding response that they can say anything they want as long as they are not mentioning any patient names and violating confidentiality.

1. Is there an ethical dilemma present in this case?
   a. Yes.
   b. No.

2. Do most institutes of higher learning have social media policies related to student conduct (on campus and off campus) that these postings may violate?
   a. No.
   b. Yes.

3. What section(s) of the ADHA Code of Ethics "Standards" may be involved in this situation?
   a. "To ourselves as professionals."
   b. "To the dental hygiene profession."
   c. "To the community and society."
   d. All of the above.
   e. None of the above.

4. A good rule of thumb when using social media is to
   a. remember that all digital communications leave a footprint
   b. never discuss nondental situations
   c. only include people who share your values
   d. attend to all of the above
   e. attend to none of the above

Testlet 8

Robert, a longstanding patient of dental hygienist Deirdre, asks to speak with her privately in her operatory. Robert closes the door and tells Deirdre that he is positive for HIV/AIDS and trusts that this information will be kept completely confidential. He is afraid that if other office members are informed, they will treat him differently and be uncomfortable with him. He was recently referred for the removal of his third molars to a local oral surgeon, and he specifically asked not to tell the surgeon about this condition. He states that he will decide if and when to tell anyone else.

1. What is the prima facie principle that Deirdre must honor?
   a. Autonomy.
   b. Beneficence.
   c. Nonmaleficence.
   d. Justice.
   e. Veracity.

2. What is the principle that the patient is basing his request on?
   a. Autonomy.
   b. Beneficence.
   c. Confidentiality.
   d. Justice.
   e. Veracity.

3. What might the dental hygienist need to treat a patient with HIV/AIDS?
   a. T-cell levels.
   b. A and C.
   c. Enhanced infection control.
   d. All of the above.
   e. Consultation with the medical provider.

4. Is there an ethical mandate to accurately record the patient's status in the patient record?
   a. Yes.
   b. No.

Testlet 9

Susan is a 24-year-old woman with a slight developmental delay who presents for her annual checkup with Gretchen, a dental hygienist in the office of SmileNice. Susan complains of pain in tooth number #9 during her appointment, and Gretchen asks her colleague Dr. Jefferies to look at the tooth. Dr. Jefferies takes a detailed history and during the process notices that Susan frequently looks away, fidgets with items in the examination room, and displays other behaviors that suggest significant anxiety and possibly incomplete or inaccurate disclosure of facts.

Dr. Jefferies gently queries Susan about the perceived behavior, and she eventually responds, "My mother told me not to tell you what happened, or the insurance won't pay."

After further exploration, Susan reveals that her injury occurred 3 months ago while riding her bicycle when she was hit by a car that ran a stop sign. Susan's mother has indicated they have only limited dental insurance through her work, which would cover examining and care for the tooth had it not been the result of an auto accident. Dr. Jefferies believes that Susan suffered a significant traumatic blow to the tooth and now has an acute problem from the devitalized pulp.

Barbara asks both Gretchen and Dr. Jefferies not to say "how the tooth got hurt because my Mom will be mad at me."

1. What is the main ethical issue raised in this case?
   a. Negligence.
   b. Informed refusal.
   c. Paternalism.
   d. Veracity.

2. This case presents issues that may be
   a. unethical
   b. illegal
   c. grounds for malpractice
   d. all of the above
   e. none of the above

3. Susan's anxiety and demeanor may cause the dental health professionals to consider
   a. referral to another care provider
   b. referral to a free clinic
   c. discussion with Susan's mother
   d. clarification with insurance carriers

Testlet 10

As Laura, a dental hygienist, was seating her long-time patient Mrs. Johnson, she noticed that the 80-year-old seemed slower and unsure of herself. During the routine recall appointment, Mrs. Johnson talked about how proud she was of her four grandchildren, especially Sammy, who was the apple of her eye. Mrs. Johnson's oral health is excellent, and when asked what type of toothbrush she is using, she smiles and cannot remember which brand. Laura and her patient laugh over this, saying how easily details slip away. After the appointment, Laura asks the patient for the name of the favorite grandchild she had mentioned. The patient appears a bit confused by the question and looks at Laura in a distracted manner. This upsets Laura as she and Mrs. Johnson have known each other for years and their families are close friends.

1. The issue that Laura may be facing here is:
   a. paternalism
   b. lack of capacity
   c. lack of veracity
   d. informed refusal

2. The dental hygienist may discuss Mrs. Johnson's oral health care with:
   a. a family member
   b. the primary care physician
   c. a surrogate decision maker
   d. all of the above

3. It is legally necessary to complete a mental and physical evaluation before proceeding with dental treatment on an elderly patient.
   a. True.
   b. False.

4. What communication strategy could the dental hygienist use in dealing with elderly patients like Mrs. Johnson?
   a. Ignore inaccurate statements.
   b. Focus on verbal and nonverbal comprehension cues.
   c. Challenge the patient's vague ideas for clarity.
   d. Speak in loud, simple sentences.

ANSWERS TO TESTLET QUESTIONS

Testlet 1

1. **d**
2. **c**
3. **b**
4. **b**

Testlet 2

1. **b**
2. **a**
3. **d**
4. **b**

Testlet 3

1. **a**
2. **d**
3. **b**
4. **a**

Testlet 4

1. **d**
2. **e**
3. **e**

Testlet 5

1. **b**
2. **d**
3. **d**

Testlet 6

1. **a**
2. **e**
3. **d**

Testlet 7

1. **a**
2. **b**
3. **a**
4. **a**

Testlet 8

1. **a**
2. **c**
3. **e**
4. **a**

Testlet 9

1. **d**
2. **d**
3. **c**

Testlet 10

1. **b**
2. **d**
3. **b**
4. **b**

Appendix A

American Dental Association Principles of Ethics and Code of Professional Conduct

With Official Advisory Opinions Revised to November 2020

ADA American Dental Association®

Contents

I. INTRODUCTION

The dental profession holds a special position of trust within society. As a consequence, society affords the profession certain privileges that are not available to members of the public-at-large. In return, the profession makes a commitment to society that its members will adhere to high ethical standards of conduct. These standards are embodied in the *ADA Principles of Ethics and Code of Professional Conduct (ADA Code)*. The *ADA Code* is, in effect, a written expression of the obligations arising from the implied contract between the dental profession and society.

Members of the ADA voluntarily agree to abide by the *ADA Code* as a condition of membership in the Association. They recognize that continued public trust in the dental profession is based on the commitment of individual dentists to high ethical standards of conduct.

The *ADA Code* has three main components: The Principles of Ethics, the Code of Professional Conduct and the Advisory Opinions.

The **Principles of Ethics** are the aspirational goals of the profession. They provide guidance and offer justification for the *Code of Professional Conduct* and the *Advisory Opinions*. There are five fundamental principles that form the foundation of the *ADA Code:* patient autonomy, nonmaleficence, beneficence, justice and veracity. Principles can overlap each other as well as compete with each other for priority.

More than one principle can justify a given element of the *Code of Professional Conduct*. Principles may at times need to be balanced against each other, but, otherwise, they are the profession's firm guideposts.

The **Code of Professional Conduct** is an expression of specific types of conduct that are either required or prohibited. The *Code of Professional Conduct* is a product of the ADA's legislative system. All elements of the *Code of Professional Conduct* result from resolutions that are adopted by the ADA's House of Delegates. The *Code of Professional Conduct* is binding on members of the ADA, and violations may result in disciplinary action.

The **Advisory Opinions** are interpretations that apply the *Code of Professional Conduct* to specific fact situations. They are adopted by the ADA's Council on Ethics, Bylaws and Judicial Affairs to provide guidance to the membership on how the Council might interpret the *Code of Professional Conduct* in a disciplinary proceeding.

The *ADA Code* is an evolving document and by its very nature cannot be a complete articulation of all ethical obligations. The *ADA Code* is the result of an on-going dialogue between the dental profession and society, and as such, is subject to continuous review.

Although ethics and the law are closely related, they are not the same. Ethical obligations may – and often do – exceed legal duties. In resolving any ethical problem not explicitly covered by the *ADA Code*, dentists should consider the ethical principles, the patient's needs and interests, and any applicable laws.

II. PREAMBLE

The American Dental Association calls upon dentists to follow high ethical standards which have the benefit of the patient as their primary goal. In recognition of this goal, the education and training of a dentist has resulted in society affording to the profession the privilege and obligation of self-government. To fulfill this privilege, these high ethical standards should be adopted and practiced throughout the dental school educational process and subsequent professional career.

The Association believes that dentists should possess not only knowledge, skill and technical competence but also those traits of character that foster adherence to ethical principles. Qualities of honesty, compassion, kindness, integrity, fairness and charity are part of the ethical education of a dentist and practice of dentistry and help to define the true professional. As such, each dentist should share in providing advocacy to and care of the underserved. It is urged that the dentist meet this goal, subject to individual circumstances.

The ethical dentist strives to do that which is right and good. The *ADA Code* is an instrument to help the dentist in this quest.

III. PRINCIPLES, CODE OF PROFESSIONAL CONDUCT AND ADVISORY OPINIONS

Section 1 Principle: Patient Autonomy ("self-governance")

The dentist has a duty to respect the patient's rights to self-determination and confidentiality.

This principle expresses the concept that professionals have a duty to treat the patient according to the patient's desires, within the bounds of accepted treatment, and to protect the patient's confidentiality. Under this principle, the dentist's primary obligations include involving patients in treatment decisions in a meaningful way, with due consideration being given to the patient's needs, desires and abilities, and safeguarding the patient's privacy.

CODE OF PROFESSIONAL CONDUCT

1.A. Patient Involvement

The dentist should inform the patient of the proposed treatment, and any reasonable alternatives, in a manner that allows the patient to become involved in treatment decisions.

1.B. Patient Records

Dentists are obliged to safeguard the confidentiality of patient records. Dentists shall maintain patient records in a manner consistent with the protection of the welfare of the patient. Upon request of a patient or another dental practitioner, dentists shall provide any information in accordance with applicable law that will be beneficial for the future treatment of that patient.

Advisory Opinions

1.B.1. Furnishing Copies of Records

A dentist has the ethical obligation on request of either the patient or the patient's new dentist to furnish in accordance with applicable law, either gratuitously or for nominal cost, such dental records or copies or summaries of them, including dental X-rays or copies of them, as will be beneficial for the future treatment of that patient. This obligation exists whether or not the patient's account is paid in full.

1.B.2. Confidentiality of Patient Records

The dominant theme in Code Section l.B is the protection of the confidentiality of a patient's records. The statement in this section that relevant information in the records should be released to another dental practitioner assumes that the dentist requesting the information is the patient's present dentist. There may be circumstances where the former dentist has an ethical obligation to inform the present dentist of certain facts. Code Section 1.B assumes that the dentist releasing relevant information is acting in accordance with applicable law. Dentists should be aware that the laws of the various jurisdictions in the United States are not uniform and some confidentiality laws appear to prohibit the transfer of pertinent information, such as HIV seropositivity. Absent certain knowledge that the laws of the dentist's jurisdiction permit the forwarding of this information, a dentist should obtain the patient's written permission before forwarding health records which contain information of a sensitive nature, such as HIV seropositivity, chemical dependency or sexual preference. If it is necessary for a treating dentist to consult with another dentist or physician with respect to the patient, and the circumstances do not permit the patient to remain anonymous, the treating dentist should seek the permission of the patient prior to the release of data from the patient's records to the consulting practitioner. If the patient refuses, the treating dentist should then contemplate obtaining legal advice regarding the termination of the dentist-patient relationship.

Section 2 Principle: Nonmaleficence ("Do No Harm")

The dentist has a duty to refrain from harming the patient.

This principle expresses the concept that professionals have a duty to protect the patient from harm. Under this principle, the dentist's primary obligations include keeping knowledge and skills current, knowing one's own limitations and when to refer to a specialist or other professional, and knowing when and under what circumstances delegation of patient care to auxiliaries is appropriate.

CODE OF PROFESSIONAL CONDUCT

2.A. Education

The privilege of dentists to be accorded professional status rests primarily in the knowledge, skill and experience with which they serve their patients and society. All dentists, therefore, have the obligation of keeping their knowledge and skill current.

2.B. Consultation and Referral

Dentists shall be obliged to seek consultation, if possible, whenever the welfare of patients will be safeguarded or advanced by utilizing those who have special skills, knowledge, and experience. When patients visit or are referred to specialists or consulting dentists for consultation:

1. The specialists or consulting dentists upon completion of their care shall return the patient, unless the patient expressly reveals a different preference, to the referring dentist, or, if none, to the dentist of record for future care.
2. The specialists shall be obliged when there is no referring dentist and upon a completion of their treatment to inform patients when there is a need for further dental care.

Advisory Opinion

2.B.1. Second Opinions

A dentist who has a patient referred by a third party[1] for a "second opinion" regarding a diagnosis or treatment plan recommended by the patient's treating dentist should render the requested second opinion in accordance with this *Code of Ethics*. In the interest of the patient being afforded quality care, the dentist rendering the second opinion should not have a vested interest in the ensuing recommendation.

2.C. Use of Auxiliary Personnel

Dentists shall be obliged to protect the health of their patients by only assigning to qualified auxiliaries those duties which can be legally delegated. Dentists shall be further obliged to prescribe and supervise the patient care provided by all auxiliary personnel working under their direction.

2.D. Personal Impairment

It is unethical for a dentist to practice while abusing controlled substances, alcohol or other chemical agents which impair the ability to practice. All dentists have an ethical obligation to urge chemically impaired colleagues to seek treatment. Dentists with first-hand knowledge that a colleague is practicing dentistry when so impaired have an ethical responsibility to report such evidence to the professional assistance committee of a dental society.

Advisory Opinion

2.D.1. Ability to Practice

A dentist who contracts any disease or becomes impaired in any way that might endanger patients or dental staff shall, with consultation and advice from a qualified physician or other authority, limit the activities of practice to those areas that do not endanger patients or dental staff. A dentist who has been advised to limit the activities of his or her practice should monitor the aforementioned disease or impairment and make additional limitations to the activities of the dentist's practice, as indicated.

2.E. Postexposure, Bloodborne Pathogens

All dentists, regardless of their bloodborne pathogen status, have an ethical obligation to immediately inform any patient who may have been exposed to blood or other potentially infectious material in the dental office of the need for postexposure evaluation and follow-up and to immediately refer the patient to a qualified health care practitioner who can provide postexposure services. The dentist's ethical obligation in the event of an exposure incident extends to providing information concerning the dentist's own bloodborne pathogen status to the evaluating health care practitioner, if the dentist is the source individual, and to submitting to testing that will assist in the evaluation of the patient. If a staff member or other third person is the source individual, the dentist should encourage that person to cooperate as needed for the patient's evaluation.

2.F. Patient Abandonment

Once a dentist has undertaken a course of treatment, the dentist should not discontinue that treatment without giving the patient adequate notice and the opportunity to obtain the services of another dentist. Care should be taken that the patient's oral health is not jeopardized in the process.

2.G. Personal Relationships with Patients

Dentists should avoid interpersonal relationships that could impair their professional judgment or risk the possibility of exploiting the confidence placed in them by a patient.

Section 3 Principle: Beneficence ("Do Good")

The dentist has a duty to promote the patient's welfare.

This principle expresses the concept that professionals have a duty to act for the benefit of others. Under this principle, the dentist's primary obligation is service to the patient and the public-at-large. The most important aspect of this obligation is the competent and timely delivery of dental care within the bounds of clinical circumstances presented by the patient, with due consideration being given to the needs, desires and values of the patient. The same ethical considerations apply whether the dentist engages in fee-for-service, managed care or some other practice arrangement. Dentists may choose to enter into contracts governing the provision of care to a group of patients; however, contract obligations do not excuse dentists from their ethical duty to put the patient's welfare first.

CODE OF PROFESSIONAL CONDUCT

3.A. Community Service

Since dentists have an obligation to use their skills, knowledge and experience for the improvement of the dental health of the public and are encouraged to be leaders in their community, dentists in such service shall conduct themselves in such a manner as to maintain or elevate the esteem of the profession.

Advisory Opinion

3.A.1. Elective and Non-Emergent Procedures During a Public Health Emergency

Dentists have ethical obligations to provide care for patients and also serve the public at large. Typically, these obligations are interrelated. Dentists are able to provide oral health care for patients according to the patient's desires and wishes, so long as the treatment is within the scope of what is deemed acceptable care without causing the patient harm or impacting the public. During public health crises or emergencies, however, the dentist's ethical obligation to the public may supersede the dentist's ethical obligations to individual patients. This may occur, for example, when a communicable disease causes individual patients who undergo treatment and/or the public to be exposed to elevated health risks. During the time of a public health emergency, therefore, dentists should balance the competing ethical obligations to individual patients and the public. If, for example, a patient requests an elective or non-emergent procedure during a public health crisis, the dentist should weigh the risk to the patient and the public from performing that procedure during the public health emergency, postponing such treatment if, in the dentist's judgment, the risk of harm to the patient and/or the public is elevated and cannot be suitably mitigated. If, however, the patient presents with an urgent or emergent condition necessitating treatment to prevent or eliminate infection or to preserve the structure and function of teeth or orofacial hard and soft tissues, the weighing of the dentist's competing ethical obligations may result in moving forward with the treatment of the patient.

3.B. Government of a Profession

Every profession owes society the responsibility to regulate itself. Such regulation is achieved largely through the influence of the professional societies. All dentists, therefore, have the dual obligation of making themselves a part of a professional society and of observing its rules of ethics.

3.C. Research and Development

Dentists have the obligation of making the results and benefits of their investigative efforts available to all when they are useful in safeguarding or promoting the health of the public.

3.D. Patents and Copyrights

Patents and copyrights may be secured by dentists provided that such patents and copyrights shall not be used to restrict research or practice.

3.E. Abuse and Neglect

Dentists shall be obliged to become familiar with the signs of abuse and neglect and to report suspected cases to the proper authorities, consistent with state laws.

Advisory Opinion

3.E.1 Reporting Abuse and Neglect

The public and the profession are best served by dentists who are familiar with identifying the signs of abuse and neglect and knowledgeable about the appropriate intervention resources for all populations.

A dentist's ethical obligation to identify and report the signs of abuse and neglect is, at a minimum, to be consistent with a dentist's legal obligation in the jurisdiction where the dentist practices. Dentists, therefore, are ethically obliged to identify and report suspected cases of abuse and neglect to the same extent as they are legally obliged to do so in the jurisdiction where they practice. Dentists have a concurrent ethical obligation to respect an adult patient's right to self-determination and confidentiality and to promote the welfare of all patients. Care should be exercised to respect the wishes of an adult patient who asks that a suspected case of abuse and/or neglect not be reported, where such a report is not mandated by law. With the patient's permission, other possible solutions may be sought.

Dentists should be aware that jurisdictional laws vary in their definitions of abuse and neglect, in their reporting requirements and the extent to which immunity is granted to good faith reporters. The variances may raise potential legal and other risks that should be considered, while keeping in mind the duty to put the welfare of the patient first. Therefore a dentist's ethical obligation to identify and report suspected cases of abuse and neglect can vary from one jurisdiction to another.

Dentists are ethically obligated to keep current their knowledge of both identifying abuse and neglect and reporting it in the jurisdiction(s) where they practice.

3.F. Professional Demeanor in the Workplace

Dentists have the obligation to provide a workplace environment that supports respectful and collaborative relationships for all those involved in oral health care.

Advisory Opinion

3.F.1 Disruptive Behavior in the Workplace

Dentists are the leaders of the oral healthcare team. As such, their behavior in the workplace is instrumental in establishing and maintaining a practice environment that supports the mutual respect, good communication, and high levels of collaboration among team members required to optimize the quality of patient care provided. Dentists who engage in disruptive behavior in the workplace risk undermining professional relationships among team members, decreasing the quality of patient care provided, and undermining the public's trust and confidence in the profession.

Section 4 Principle: Justice ("Fairness")

The dentist has a duty to treat people fairly.

This principle expresses the concept that professionals have a duty to be fair in their dealings with patients, colleagues and society. Under this principle, the dentist's primary obligations include dealing with people justly and delivering dental care without prejudice. In its broadest sense, this principle expresses the concept that the dental profession should actively seek allies throughout society on specific activities that will help improve access to care for all.

CODE OF PROFESSIONAL CONDUCT

4.A. Patient Selection

While dentists, in serving the public, may exercise reasonable discretion in selecting patients for their practices, dentists shall not refuse to accept patients into their practice or deny dental service to patients because of the patient's race, creed, color, gender, sexual orientation, gender identity, national origin or disability.

Advisory Opinion

4.A.1. Patients with Disabilities or Bloodborne Pathogens

As is the case with all patients, when considering the treatment of patients with a physical, intellectual or developmental disability or disabilities, including patients infected with Human Immunodeficiency Virus, Hepatitis B Virus, Hepatitis C Virus or another bloodborne pathogen, or are otherwise medically compromised, the individual dentist should determine if he or she has the need of another's skills, knowledge, equipment or expertise, and if so, consultation or referral pursuant to Section 2.B hereof is indicated. Decisions regarding the type of dental treatment provided, or referrals made or suggested, should be made on the same basis as they are made with other patients. The dentist should also determine, after consultation with the patient's physician, if appropriate, if the patient's health status would be significantly compromised by the provision of dental treatment.

4.B. Emergency Service

Dentists shall be obliged to make reasonable arrangements for the emergency care of their patients of record. Dentists shall be obliged when consulted in an emergency by patients not of record to make reasonable arrangements for emergency care. If treatment is provided, the dentist, upon completion of treatment, is obliged to return the patient to his or her regular dentist unless the patient expressly reveals a different preference.

4.C. Justifiable Criticism

Dentists shall be obliged to report to the appropriate reviewing agency as determined by the local component or constituent society instances of gross or continual faulty treatment by other dentists. Patients should be informed of their present oral health status without disparaging comment about prior services. Dentists issuing a public statement with respect to the profession shall have a reasonable basis to believe that the comments made are true.

Advisory Opinion

4.C.1. Meaning of "Justifiable"

Patients are dependent on the expertise of dentists to know their oral health status. Therefore, when informing a patient of the status of his or her oral health, the dentist should exercise care that the comments made are truthful, informed and justifiable. This should, if possible, involve consultation with the previous treating dentist(s), in accordance with applicable law, to determine under what circumstances and conditions the

treatment was performed. A difference of opinion as to preferred treatment should not be communicated to the patient in a manner which would unjustly imply mistreatment. There will necessarily be cases where it will be difficult to determine whether the comments made are justifiable. Therefore, this section is phrased to address the discretion of dentists and advises against unknowing or unjustifiable disparaging statements against another dentist. However, it should be noted that, where comments are made which are not supportable and therefore unjustified, such comments can be the basis for the institution of a disciplinary proceeding against the dentist making such statements.

4.D. Expert Testimony

Dentists may provide expert testimony when that testimony is essential to a just and fair disposition of a judicial or administrative action.

Advisory Opinion

4.D.1. Contingent Fees

It is unethical for a dentist to agree to a fee contingent upon the favorable outcome of the litigation in exchange for testifying as a dental expert.

4.E. Rebates and Split Fees

Dentists shall not accept or tender "rebates" or "split fees."

Advisory Opinion

4.E.1. Split Fees in Advertising and Marketing Services

The prohibition against a dentist's accepting or tendering rebates or split fees applies to business dealings between dentists and any third party, not just other dentists. Thus, a dentist who pays for advertising or marketing services by sharing a specified portion of the professional fees collected from prospective or actual patients with the vendor providing the advertising or marketing services is engaged in fee splitting. The prohibition against fee splitting is also applicable to the marketing of dental treatments or procedures via "social coupons" if the business arrangement between the dentist and the concern providing the marketing services for that treatment or those procedures allows the issuing company to collect the fee from the prospective patient, retain a defined percentage or portion of the revenue collected as payment for the coupon marketing service provided to the dentist and remit to the dentist the remainder of the amount collected.

Dentists should also be aware that the laws or regulations in their jurisdictions may contain provisions that impact the division of revenue collected from prospective patients between a dentist and a third party to pay for advertising or marketing services.

Section 5 Principle: Veracity ("Truthfulness")

The dentist has a duty to communicate truthfully.

This principle expresses the concept that professionals have a duty to be honest and trustworthy in their dealings with people. Under this principle, the dentist's primary obligations include respecting the position of trust inherent in the dentist-patient relationship, communicating truthfully and without deception, and maintaining intellectual integrity.

CODE OF PROFESSIONAL CONDUCT

5.A. Representation of Care

Dentists shall not represent the care being rendered to their patients in a false or misleading manner.

Advisory Opinions

5.A.1. Dental Amalgam and other Restorative Materials

Based on current scientific data, the ADA has determined that the removal of amalgam restorations from the non-allergic patient for the alleged purpose of removing toxic substances from the body, when such treatment is performed solely at the recommendation of the dentist, is improper and unethical. The same principle of veracity applies to the dentist's recommendation concerning the removal of any dental restorative material.

5.A.2. Unsubstantiated Representations

A dentist who represents that dental treatment or diagnostic techniques recommended or performed by the dentist has the capacity to diagnose, cure or alleviate diseases, infections or other conditions, when such representations are not based upon accepted scientific knowledge or research, is acting unethically.

5.B. Representation of Fees

Dentists shall not represent the fees being charged for providing care in a false or misleading manner.

Advisory Opinions

5.B.1. Waiver of Copayment

A dentist who accepts a third party[1] payment under a copayment plan as payment in full without disclosing to the third party[1] that the patient's payment portion will not be collected, is engaged in overbilling. The essence of this ethical impropriety is deception and misrepresentation; an overbilling dentist makes it appear to the third party[1] that the charge to the patient for services rendered is higher than it actually is.

5.B.2. Overbilling

It is unethical for a dentist to increase a fee to a patient solely because the patient is covered under a dental benefits plan.

5.B.3. Fee Differential

The fee for a patient without dental benefits shall be considered a dentist's full fee.[2] This is the fee that should be represented to all benefit carriers regardless of any negotiated fee discount. Payments accepted by a dentist under a governmentally funded program, a component or constituent dental society-sponsored access program, or a participating agreement entered into under a program with a third party shall not be considered or construed as evidence of overbilling in determining whether a charge to a patient, or to another third party[1] in behalf of a patient not covered under any of the aforecited programs constitutes overbilling **under** this section of the *Code*.

5.B.4. Treatment Dates

A dentist who submits a claim form to a third party[1] reporting incorrect treatment dates for the purpose of assisting a patient in obtaining benefits under a dental plan, which benefits would otherwise be disallowed, is engaged in making an unethical, false or misleading representation to such third party.[1]

5.B.5. Dental Procedures

A dentist who incorrectly describes on a third party[1] claim form a dental procedure in order to receive a greater payment or reimbursement or incorrectly makes a non-covered procedure appear to be a covered procedure on such a claim form is engaged in making an unethical, false or misleading representation to such third party.[1]

5.B.6. Unnecessary Services

A dentist who recommends or performs unnecessary dental services or procedures is engaged in unethical conduct. The dentist's ethical obligation in this matter applies regardless of the type of practice arrangement or contractual obligations in which he or she provides patient care.

5.C. Disclosure of Conflict of Interest

A dentist who presents educational or scientific information in an article, seminar or other program shall disclose to the readers or participants any monetary or other special interest the dentist may have with a company whose products are promoted or endorsed in the presentation. Disclosure shall be made in any promotional material and in the presentation itself.

5.D. Devices and Therapeutic Methods

Except for formal investigative studies, dentists shall be obliged to prescribe, dispense, or promote only those devices, drugs and other agents whose complete formulae are available to the dental profession. Dentists shall have the further obligation of not holding out as exclusive any device, agent, method or technique if that representation would be false or misleading in any material respect.

Advisory Opinions

5.D.1. Reporting Adverse Reactions

A dentist who suspects the occurrence of an adverse reaction to a drug or dental device has an obligation to communicate that information to the broader medical and dental community, including, in the case of a serious adverse event, the Food and Drug Administration (FDA).

5.D.2. Marketing or Sale of Products or Procedures

Dentists who, in the regular conduct of their practices, engage in or employ auxiliaries in the marketing or sale of products or procedures to their patients must take care not to exploit the trust inherent in the dentist-patient relationship for their own financial gain. Dentists should not induce their patients to purchase products or undergo procedures by misrepresenting the product's value, the necessity of the procedure or the dentist's professional expertise in recommending the product or procedure.

In the case of a health-related product, it is not enough for the dentist to rely on the manufacturer's or distributor's representations about the product's safety and efficacy. The dentist has an independent obligation to inquire into the truth and accuracy of such claims and verify that they are founded on accepted scientific knowledge or research.

Dentists should disclose to their patients all relevant information the patient needs to make an informed purchase decision, including whether the product is available elsewhere and whether there are any financial incentives for the dentist to recommend the product that would not be evident to the patient.

5.E. Professional Announcement

In order to properly serve the public, dentists should represent themselves in a manner that contributes to the esteem of the profession. Dentists should not misrepresent their training and competence in any way that would be false or misleading in any material respect.[3]

5.F. Advertising

Although any dentist may advertise, no dentist shall advertise or solicit patients in any form of communication in a manner that is false or misleading in any material respect.[3]

Advisory Opinions

5.F.1. Published Communications

If a dental health article, message or newsletter is published in print or electronic media under a dentist's byline to the public without making truthful disclosure of the source and authorship or is designed to give rise to questionable expectations for the purpose of inducing the public to utilize the services of the sponsoring dentist, the dentist is engaged in making a false or misleading representation to the public in a material respect.[3]

5.F.2. Examples of "False or Misleading"

The following examples are set forth to provide insight into the meaning of the term "false or misleading in a material respect."[3] These examples are not meant to be all-inclusive. Rather, by restating the concept in alternative language and giving general examples, it is hoped that the membership will gain a better understanding of the term. With this in mind, statements shall be avoided which would: a) contain a material misrepresentation of fact, b) omit a fact necessary to make the statement considered as a whole not materially misleading, c) be intended or be likely to create an unjustified expectation about results the dentist can achieve, and d) contain a material, objective representation, whether express or implied, that the advertised services are superior in quality to those of other dentists, if that representation is not subject to reasonable substantiation.

Subjective statements about the quality of dental services can also raise ethical concerns. In particular, statements of opinion may be misleading if they are not honestly held, if they misrepresent the qualifications of the holder, or the basis of the opinion, or if the patient reasonably interprets them as implied statements of fact. Such statements will be evaluated on a case by case basis, considering how patients are likely to respond to the impression made by the advertisement as a whole. The fundamental issue is whether the advertisement, taken as a whole, is false or misleading in a material respect.[3]

5.F.3. Unearned, Nonhealth Degrees

A dentist may use the title Doctor or Dentist, D.D.S., D.M.D. or any additional earned, advanced academic degrees in health service areas in an announcement to the public. The announcement of an unearned academic degree may be misleading because of the likelihood that it will indicate to the public the attainment of specialty or diplomate status.

For purposes of this advisory opinion, an unearned academic degree is one which is awarded by an educational institution not accredited by a generally recognized accrediting body or is an honorary degree.

The use of a nonhealth degree in an announcement to the public may be a representation which is misleading because the public is likely to assume that any degree announced is related to the qualifications of the dentist as a practitioner.

Some organizations grant dentists fellowship status as a token of membership in the organization or some other form of voluntary association. The use of such fellowships in advertising to the general public may be misleading because of the likelihood that it will indicate to the public attainment of education or skill in the field of dentistry.

Generally, unearned or nonhealth degrees and fellowships that designate association, rather than attainment, should be limited to scientific papers and curriculum vitae. In all instances, state law should be consulted. In any review by the council of the use of designations in advertising to the public, the council will apply the standard of whether the use of such is false or misleading in a material respect.[3]

5.F.4. Referral Services

There are two basic types of referral services for dental care: not-for-profit and the commercial. The not-for-profit is commonly organized by dental societies or community services. It is open to all qualified practitioners in the area served. A fee is sometimes charged the practitioner to be listed with the service. A fee for such referral services is for the purpose of covering the expenses of the service and has no relation to the number of patients referred. In contrast, some commercial referral services restrict access to the referral service to a limited number of dentists in a particular geographic area. Prospective patients calling the service may be referred to a single subscribing dentist in the geographic area and the respective dentist billed for each patient referred. Commercial referral services often advertise to the public stressing that there is no charge for use of the service and the patient may not be informed of the referral fee paid by the dentist. There is a connotation to such advertisements that the referral that is being made is in the nature of a public service. A dentist is allowed to pay for any advertising permitted by the *Code*, but is generally not permitted to make payments to another person or entity for the referral of a patient for professional services. While the particular facts and circumstances relating to an individual commercial referral service will vary, the council believes that the aspects outlined above for commercial referral services violate the *Code* in that it constitutes advertising which is false or misleading in a material respect and violates the prohibitions in the *Code* against fee splitting.[3]

5.F.5. Infectious Disease Test Results

An advertisement or other communication intended to solicit patients which omits a material fact or facts necessary to put the information conveyed in the advertisement in a proper context can be misleading in a material respect. A dental practice should not seek to attract patients on the basis of partial truths which create a false impression.[3]

For example, an advertisement to the public of HIV negative test results, without conveying additional information that will clarify the scientific significance of this fact contains a misleading omission. A dentist could satisfy his or her obligation under this advisory opinion to convey additional information by clearly stating in the advertisement or other communication: "This negative HIV test cannot guarantee that I am currently free of HIV."

5.F.6. Websites and Search Engine Optimization

Many dentists employ an Internet web site to announce their practices, introduce viewers to the professionals and staff in the office, describe practice philosophies and impart oral health care information to the public. Dentists may use services to increase the visibility of their web sites when consumers perform searches for dentally-related content. This technique is generally known as "search engine optimization" or "SEO." Dentists have an ethical obligation to ensure that their web sites, like their other professional announcements, are truthful and do not present information in a manner that is false and misleading in a material respect.[3] Also, any SEO techniques used in connection with a dentist's web site should comport with the ADA *Principles of Ethics and Code of Professional Conduct.*

5.G. Name of Practice

Since the name under which a dentist conducts his or her practice may be a factor in the selection process

of the patient, the use of a trade name or an assumed name that is false or misleading in any material respect is unethical. Use of the name of a dentist no longer actively associated with the practice may be continued for a period not to exceed one year.[3]

Advisory Opinion

5.G.1. Dentist Leaving Practice

Dentists leaving a practice who authorize continued use of their names should receive competent advice on the legal implications of this action. With permission of a departing dentist, his or her name may be used for more than one year, if, after the one year grace period has expired, prominent notice is provided to the public through such mediums as a sign at the office and a short statement on stationery and business cards that the departing dentist has retired from the practice.

5.H. Announcement of Specialization and Limitation of Practice

A dentist may ethically announce as a specialist to the public in any of the dental specialties recognized by the National Commission on Recognition of Dental Specialties and Certifying Boards including dental public health, endodontics, oral and maxillofacial pathology, oral and maxillofacial radiology, oral and maxillofacial surgery, orthodontics and dentofacial orthopedics, pediatric dentistry, periodontics, and prosthodontics, and in any other areas of dentistry for which specialty recognition has been granted under the standards required or recognized in the practitioner's jurisdiction, provided the dentist meets the educational requirements required for recognition as a specialist adopted by the American Dental Association or accepted in the jurisdiction in which they practice.* Dentists who choose to announce specialization

---

*In the case of the ADA, the educational requirements include successful completion of an advanced educational program accredited by the Commission on Dental Accreditation, two or more years in length, as specified by the Council on Dental Education and Licensure, or being a diplomate of an American Dental Association recognized certifying board for each specialty announced.

should use "specialist in" and shall devote a sufficient portion of their practice to the announced specialty or specialties to maintain expertise in that specialty or those specialties, Dentists whose practice is devoted exclusively to an announced specialty or specialties may announce that their practice "is limited to" that specialty or those specialties. Dentists who use their eligibility to announce as specialists to make the public believe that specialty services rendered in the dental office are being rendered by qualified specialists when such is not the case are engaged in unethical conduct. The burden of responsibility is on specialists to avoid any inference that general practitioners who are associated with specialists are qualified to announce themselves as specialists.

Advisory Opinions

5.H.1. Dual Degreed Dentists

Nothing in Section 5.H shall be interpreted to prohibit a dual degreed dentist who practices medicine or osteopathy under a valid state license from announcing to the public as a dental specialist provided the dentist meets the educational, experience and other standards set forth in the *Code* for specialty announcement and further providing that the announcement is truthful and not materially misleading.

5.H.2. Specialist Announcement of Credentials In Non-Specialty Interest Areas

A dentist who is qualified to announce specialization under this section may not announce to the public that he or she is certified or a diplomate or otherwise similarly credentialed in an area of dentistry not recognized as a specialty area by the National Commission on Recognition of Dental Specialties and Certifying Boards or by the jurisdiction in which the dentist practices unless:

1. The organization granting the credential grants certification or diplomate status based on the following: a) the dentist's successful completion of a formal, full-time advanced education program (graduate or postgraduate level) of at least 12 months' duration; and b) the dentist's training and experience; and c) successful completion of an oral and written examination based on psychometric principles; and

2. The announcement includes the following language: [Name of announced area of dental practice] is not recognized as a specialty area by the National Commission on Recognition of Dental Specialties and Certifying Boards or [the name of the jurisdiction in which the dentist practices].

Nothing in this advisory opinion affects the right of a properly qualified dentist to announce specialization in a recognized specialty area(s) or the responsibility of such dentist to maintain exclusivity in the special area(s) of dental practice announced as provided for under Section 5.H of this *Code*. Specialists shall not announce their credentials in a manner that implies specialization in a non-specialty interest area.

5.I. General Practitioner Announcement of Services

General dentists who wish to announce the services available in their practices are permitted to announce the availability of those services so long as they avoid any communications that express or imply specialization. General dentists shall also state that the services are being provided by general dentists. No dentist shall announce available services in any way that would be false or misleading in any material respect.[3]

Advisory Opinions

5.I.1. General Practitioner Announcement of Credentials in Interest Areas in General Dentistry

A general dentist may not announce to the public that he or she is certified or a diplomate or otherwise similarly credentialed in an area of dentistry not recognized as a specialty area by the National Commission on Recognition of Dental Specialties and Certifying Boards or by the jurisdiction in which the dentist practices unless:

1. The organization granting the credential grants certification or diplomate status based on the following: a) the dentist's successful completion of a formal, full-time advanced education program (graduate or postgraduate level) of at least 12 months duration; and b) the dentist's training and experience; and c) successful completion of an oral and written examination based on psychometric principles;

2. The dentist discloses that he or she is a general dentist; and

3. The announcement includes the following language: [Name of announced area of dental practice] is not recognized as a specialty area by the National Commission on Recognition of Dental Specialties and Certifying Boards or [the name of the jurisdiction in which the dentist practices].

5.I.2. Credentials in General Dentistry

General dentists may announce fellowships or other credentials earned in the area of general dentistry so long as they avoid any communications that express or imply specialization and the announcement includes the disclaimer that the dentist is a general dentist. The use of abbreviations to designate credentials shall be avoided when such use would lead the reasonable person to believe that the designation represents an academic degree, when such is not the case.

NOTES

1. A third party is any party to a dental prepayment contract that may collect premiums, assume financial risks, pay claims, and/or provide administrative services.

2. A full fee is the fee for a service that is set by the dentist, which reflects the costs of providing the procedure and the value of the dentist's professional judgment.

3. Advertising, solicitation of patients or business or other promotional activities by dentists or dental care delivery organizations shall not be considered unethical or improper, except for those promotional activities which are false or misleading in any material respect. Notwithstanding any *ADA Principles of Ethics and Code of Professional Conduct* or other standards of dentist conduct which may be differently worded, this shall be the sole standard for determining the ethical propriety of such promotional activities. Any provision of an ADA constituent or component society's code of ethics or other standard of dentist conduct relating to dentists' or dental care delivery organizations' advertising, solicitation, or other promotional ac-

tivities which is worded differently from the above standard shall be deemed to be in conflict with the *ADA Principles of Ethics and Code of Professional Conduct.*

4. Completion of three years of advanced training in oral and maxillofacial surgery or two years of advanced training in one of the other recognized dental specialties prior to 1967.

IV. INTERPRETATION AND APPLICATION OF PRINCIPLES OF ETHICS AND CODE OF PROFESSIONAL CONDUCT

The foregoing *ADA Principles of Ethics and Code of Professional Conduct* set forth the ethical duties that are binding on members of the American Dental Association. The component and constituent societies may adopt additional requirements or interpretations not in conflict with the *ADA Code.*

Anyone who believes that a member-dentist has acted unethically should bring the matter to the attention of the appropriate constituent (state) or component (local) dental society. Whenever possible, problems involving questions of ethics should be resolved at the state or local level. If a satisfactory resolution cannot be reached, the dental society may decide, after proper investigation, that the matter warrants issuing formal charges and conducting a disciplinary hearing pursuant to the procedures set forth in Chapter XI of the ADA *Bylaws* and *Governance and Organizational Manual of the American Dental Association* ("*Governance Manual*").

PRINCIPLES OF ETHICS AND CODE OF PROFESSIONAL CONDUCT, MEMBER CONDUCT POLICY AND JUDICIAL PROCEDURES. The Council on Ethics, Bylaws and Judicial Affairs reminds constituent and component societies that before a dentist can be found to have breached any ethical obligation the dentist is entitled to a fair hearing.

A member who is found guilty of unethical conduct proscribed by the *ADA Code* or code of ethics of the constituent or component society, may be placed under a sentence of censure or suspension or may be expelled from membership in the

Association. A member under a sentence of censure, suspension or expulsion has the right to appeal the decision to his or her constituent society and the ADA Council on Ethics, Bylaws and Judicial Affairs, as provided in Chapter XI of the ADA *Bylaws* and *Governance Manual*.

V. CEBJA STATEMENTS AND WHITE PAPERS

THE STATEMENTS AND WHITE PAPERS BELOW HAVE BEEN PREPARED BY CEBJA AND ARE AVAILABLE FOR VIEWING OR DOWNLOAD IN PDF FORMAT AT www.ada.org/cebjastatements:

Announcement of Credentials in General Dentistry—Last reviewed 2021

Dental Tourism—*Last reviewed 2020*

Ethical Aspects of Dental Practice Arrangements—*Last reviewed 2020*

Ethical Considerations When Using Patients in the Examination Process—*Last reviewed 2020*

The Ethics of Temporary Charitable Events—*Last reviewed 2020*

General Practitioner Announcement of Credentials in Non-Specialty Interest Areas—*Last reviewed 2019*

Gift Giving to Dentists from Patients, Colleagues and Industry—*Last reviewed 2020*

Marketing or Sale of Products or Procedures—*Last reviewed 2022*

Patient Rights and Responsibilities—*Last reviewed 2019*

Reporting Abuse and Neglect—*Last reviewed 2020*

Specialist Announcement of Credentials in Non-Specialty Interest Areas—*Last reviewed 2019*

Statement on the Ethics of the Measles Crisis—*Created 2019*

Statement Regarding the Employment of a Dentist—*Last reviewed 2018*

Treating Patients with Infectious Diseases Having Unknown Transmission Parameters—*Initial adoption 2022*

Unearned Nonhealth Degrees—*Last reviewed 2021*

VI. INDEX

ADVISORY OPINIONS ARE DESIGNATED BY THEIR RELEVANT SECTION IN PARENTHESES, e.g. (2.D.1.).

Bibliography and Suggested Readings

Acierno R, Hernandez MA, Amstadter AB, et al.: Prevalence and correlates of emotional, physical, sexual, and financial abuse, and potential neglect in the United States: The National Elder Mistreatment Study, *American Journal of Public Health* 100(2):292–297, 2010.

Adler MJ: *Aristotle for Everybody*. Bantam Books; 1978.

American Academy of Periodontology. Comprehensive periodontal therapy: A statement by the American Academy of Periodontology, *Journal of Periodontology* 82:943–949, 2011.

American Association of Dental Schools: Curriculum guidelines in dental professional ethics, *Journal of Dental Education* 53:144, 1989.

American Association of Critical Care Nurses. AACN Public Policy Position Statement: Moral Distress. Author; 2008. www.aacn.org/WD/Practice/Docs/moral_distress.pdf

American Dental Association. *Managing Patients; Informed Consent/Refusal*. ADA Center for Professional Success; 2021.

American Dental Association and FDA (US Department of Health and Human Services Public Health Service Food and Drug Administration) Dental radiographic examinations: Recommendations for patient selection and limiting radiation exposure; 2012. https://www.fda.gov/media/84818/download

American Dental Association Commission on Dental Accreditation. Accreditation Standards for Dental Hygiene Education Programs, 2020.

American Dental Association Commission on Dental Education, Dental Therapy Education Standards. https://www.ada.org/~/media/CODA/Files/dental_therapy_standards.pdf?la=en

American Dental Association Council on Ethics, Bylaws, and Judicial Affairs. ADA Principles of Ethics and Code of Professional Conduct; 2012.

American Dental Association. Glossary of Dental Administrative Terms Definition of Oral Health Literacy; 2021.

American Dental Education Association. ADEA policy statements, *Journal of Dental Education* 78:1057, 2014.

American Dental Education Association. Competencies for entry into the profession of dental hygiene; 2011. https://www.adea.org/about_adea/governance/documents/competency-docs2011.pdf

American Dental Hygienists' Association. Code of Ethics for Dental Hygienists; 2021.

American Dental Hygienists' Association. Dental Hygiene Participation in Regulation. https://www.adha.org/resources-docs/75111_Self_Regulation_by_State.pdf

American Dental Hygienists' Association. Practice Act Overview. https://oralhealthworkforce.org/resources/variation-in-dental-hygiene-scope-of-practice-by-state/

American Dental Hygienists' Association. Standards for clinical dental hygiene practice; 2016. https://www.adha.org/resources-docs/2016-Revised-Standards-for-Clinical-Dental-Hygiene-Practice.pdf

American Dental Hygienists' Association. Transforming Dental Hygiene Education and the Profession for the 21st Century. https://tenndha.com/adha-transforming-dental-hygiene-education-and-the-profession-for-the-21st-century/

American Health Information Management Association. Healthcare documentation quality assessment and management best practices; 2017. https://www.ahdionline.org/page/qa

American Psychological Association. Dictionary Definition of Cultural Sensitivity, 2021.

Anderson RM, Davidson PL, Atchison KA, et al.: Pipeline, profession, and practice program: Evaluating change in dental education, *Journal of Dental Education* 69(2):239, 2005.

Audi R: *The Cambridge Dictionary of Philosophy*, 3rd ed., 2015, Oxford University Press.

Barish NH, Barish AM: The ethical dilemma of the dental hygienist, *Journal of the American College of Dentists* 39:169, 1972.

Barstow C, Shahan B, Roberts M: Evaluating medical decision-making capacity in practice, *American Family Physician* 98(1): 40–46, 2018.

Beauchamp TL, Childress J: *Principles of Biomedical Ethics*, 8th ed., 2019, Oxford University Press.

Bebeau MJ: Teaching ethics in dentistry, *Journal of Dental Education* 49:236, 1985.

Bebeau MJ, Born DO, Ozar DT: The development of a professional role orientation inventory, *Journal of the American College of Dentists* 60(2):27, 1993.

Bebeau MJ, Thoma SJ: The impact of a dental ethics curriculum on moral reasoning, *Journal of Dental Education* 58(9):684, 1994.

Bebeau MJ, Rest JR, Narváez DF: Beyond the promise: a perspective for research in moral education, *Education Research and Reviews* 28(4):18, 1999.

Bebeau MJ, Kahn J: Ethical issues in community dental health. In Gluck GM, Morganstein WM, editors: *Jong's Community Dental Health*, 5th ed. Mosby; 2002, 425–445.

Beemsterboer PL: Competency in allied dental education, *Journal of Dental Education* 11:19, 1994.

Beemsterboer PL: Developing an ethic of access to care in dentistry, *Journal of Dental Education* 70(11):212, 2006.

Beemsterboer PL, Odom JG, Pate TD, et al.: Issues of academic integrity in U.S. dental schools, *Journal of Dental Education* 64:833, 2000.

Beemsterboer PL, Odom J: Ethical principles in clinical decision making, *Journal of the California Dental Hygienists' Association* 17(1):7–9, 12, 2001.

Beemsterboer PL, Chiodo GT: Care versus commerce: A challenge to professional integrity? *Journal of the California Dental Association*, July 2013.

Beemsterboer PL, Chiodo GT: *Allegations of overtreatment in dentistry: A perpetual issue? Membership Matters.* Oregon Dental Association; September 2013.

Beemsterboer PL, Chiodo GC: The foundation of integrity, *Dimensions of Dental Hygiene* 12:1, 2014.

Benjamin M, Curtis J: *Ethics in Nursing*, 2nd ed. Oxford University Press; 1986.

Biddington WR: The dental policy perspective, *Journal of the American College of Dentists* 57:20, 1990.

Biddington WR, Nash DA: A person within a community of persons, *Journal of the American College of Dentists* 51:12, 1984.

Black's Law Dictionary, 10th ed. Thomson West Publishing Company; 2014.

Brennan M, et al.: *Ethics and Law for the Dental Team.* PasTest Ltd; 2006.

Brueck MK, Sulmasy DP: *The rule of double effect a tool for moral deliberation in practice and policy.* Center for Bioethics Harvard Medical School; 2020. https://bioethics.hms.edu/journal/rule-double-effect

Campbell CS, Rodgers VC: The normative principles of dental ethics. In Weinstein BD, editor: *Dental Ethics.* Lea & Febiger; 1993.

Carr MP: Lawsuit pending against Florida dental hygienist, *Dimensions of Dental Hygiene*, 2018. https://dimensionsofdentalhygiene.com/lawsuit-pending-against-florida-dental-hygienist/

Carr MP, Kearney R: Standards for patient scheduling, *Dimensions of Dental Hygiene* 15(6):54, 2017. https://dimensionsofdentalhygiene.com/article/standards-patient-scheduling/

Census Bureau Report. Projections of the Size and Composition of the U.S. Population: 2014 to 2060 Population Estimates and Projections, Release Number: CB15-TPS, March 16, 2015.

Catalanotto FA: In defense of dental therapy: An evidence-based workforce approach to improving access to care, *Journal of Dental Education* 83(2 Suppl):S7–S15, 2019. doi:10.21815/JDE.019.036.

Chambers DW: Toward a competency-based curriculum, *Journal of Dental Education* 57:790, 1993.

Chambers DW: The professions, *Journal of the American College of Dentists* 71(4):57, 2004.

Chambers DW: Access denied: Invalid password, *Journal of Dental Education* 70(11):1146, 2006.

Chambers DW: Basic oral health needs: A public priority, *Journal of Dental Education* 70(11):1159, 2006.

Chambers DW: Moral communities, *Journal of Dental Education* 70(11):1226, 2006.

Chi MT, Glaser R, Farr M: *The Nature of Expertise.* Lawrence Erlbaum; 1988.

Chi DL, Lenaker D, Mancl L, Dunbar M, Babb M: Dental therapists linked to improved dental outcomes for Alaska Native communities in the Yukon-Kuskokwim Delta, *Journal of Public Health Dentistry* 78(2):175–182, 2018. doi:10.1111/jphd.12263.

Childress JF: *Who Should Decide? Paternalism in Health Care.* Oxford University Press; 1982.

Christie CR, Bowen DM, Paarmann CS: Curriculum evaluation of ethical reasoning and professional responsibility, *Journal of Dental Education* 67:55, 2003.

Christie CR, Bowen DM, Paarmann CS: Effectiveness of faculty training to enhance clinical evaluation of student competence in ethical reasoning and professionalism, *Journal of Dental Education* 71:1048, 2007.

Cianflone D, Riccelli AE: Ethical considerations for dental hygienists in private practice settings, *Journal of Dental Hygiene* 65:277, 1991.

Corley MC: Nurse moral distress: a proposed theory and research agenda. *Nursing Ethics* 9:636, 2002.

Corsino BV, Patthoff DE: The ethical and practical aspects of acceptance and universal patient acceptance, *Journal of Dental Education* 70(11):1198, 2006.

Crall JJ: Access to oral health care: Professional and societal considerations, *Journal of Dental Education* 70(11):1133, 2006.

Darby M, Walsh M: *Dental Hygiene Theory and Practice*, 4th ed. Saunders Elsevier; 2015.

Davidson JA: *Legal and Ethical Considerations for Dental Hygienists and Assistants.* Mosby; 2000.

DePaola DP: Beyond the university: leadership for the common good. American Association of Dental Schools, 75th Anniversary Summit Conference, Discussion, Papers, and Proceedings, Washington, DC, October 12–13, 1998.

Dharamsi S: Building moral communities? First, do no harm, *Journal of Dental Education* 70(11):1235, 2006.

Dharamsi S, MacEntee M: Dentistry and distributive justice, *Social Science & Medicine* 55:323, 2002.

Donabedian A: Evaluating the quality of medical care, *Milbank Memorial Fund Quarterly* 44(3):166–206, 1966. Reprinted in Milbank Quarterly. 83(4):691–729, 2005.

Dreyfus HL, Dreyfus SE: *Mind Over Machine.* The Free Press; 1986.

Edelstein BL: Disparities in oral health and access to care: Findings of national surveys, *Ambulatory Pediatrics* 2(Suppl 2):141, 2002.

Edge RS, Groves JR: *Ethics of Health Care: A Guide for Clinical Practice*, 3rd ed. Delmar; 2006.

Faden RR, King NM, Beauchamp TL: *A History and Theory of Informed Consent.* Oxford University Press; 1986.

Formicola AJ, et al.: Interprofessional education in U.S. and Canadian dental schools: An ADEA Team Study Group report, *Journal of Dental Education* 76(9):1250–1268, 2012.

Fisher-Owens SA, Lukefahr JL, Tate AR: Oral and dental aspects of child abuse and neglect, *Pediatric Dentistry* 39(4):278–283, 2017.

Francoeur RT: *Biomedical Ethics: A Guide to Decision Making.* John Wiley Sons; 1983.

Frankena WK: *Ethics*, 2nd ed. Prentice-Hall; 1963.

Garcia RI: Addressing oral health disparities in diverse populations, *Journal of the American Dental Association* 136:1210, 2005.

Garetto LP, Yoder KM: Basic oral health needs: A professional priority? *Journal of Dental Education* 70(11):1166, 2006.

Gaston MA, Brown DM, Waring MB: Survey of ethical issues in dental hygiene, *Journal of Dental Hygiene* 64:216, 1990.

Gilligan C: *In a Different Voice.* Harvard University Press; 1982.